SVALI

THE SVALI CHRONICLES
BREAKING FREE FROM MIND CONTROL
TESTIMONY OF AN EX-ILLUMINATI

ℴMNIA VERITAS.

SVALI

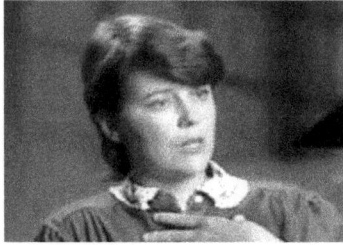

THE SVALI CHRONICLES

BREAKING FREE FROM MIND CONTROL
TESTIMONY OF AN EX-ILLUMINATI

Edited and published by

OMNIA VERITAS LTD

⊘MNIA VERITAS.

www.omnia-veritas.com

© Copyright Omnia Veritas Limited - 2023

ABOUT THE AUTHOR

Hello, my name is Svali. My whole family and I were part of a cult group until we broke free several years ago. I was a programmer in the cult, and now I want to share the knowledge I have to help others.

It is possible to break free from the abuse of a cult if one is involved. It is a long and heartbreaking process, but one that is worth the effort. In the articles I'm about to offer, I hope to help survivors of cult abuse find tools to help them on their journey to freedom.

For the past year and a half, I have been a consultant to an online survivor group that helps people cope with and break free from cult programs. I myself have been in therapy for ritual abuse and DID[1] for the past nine years, the last five of which have been marked by recent cult abuse.

I am also a writer and a registered nurse. I currently work as a diabetes educator in Texas, 20 hours a week.

I also self-published a book on how to break free from cult programming, which several experts in the field have said contains "invaluable information" for survivors of ritual abuse.

Last year, my ex-husband and two children were freed from cult abuse. My children live with me while my husband works on his recovery. They all have dissociative identity disorder (formerly known as multiple personality disorder), which makes life at home interesting! I am currently married to my second husband, who also recovered from DID and came out of the cult five years ago.

---

[1] Dissociative Identity Disorder.

EQUIPMENT FREQUENTLY USED BY TRAINERS

I t can be helpful for therapists to be aware of the equipment used by trainers. If their client describes these items, which may seem very sophisticated, they should believe them. The cult has become very technologically advanced.

Training Room: The average training room is a neutral colored room with walls painted in dull gray, white or beige. Some may be painted in different colors as part of a color code. They are often located in secret underground rooms or in the basements of large private residences, and are accessed from the main building through a covered door. Improvised training rooms may be set up during outdoor military exercises in covered canvas tents.

Trainers: The Illuminati have a rule that there must always be at least two trainers working with a person. This prevents one trainer from being too strict or too permissive, or from developing too close a bond with the subject; the watchful eye of the other trainer prevents this. Younger trainers are paired with older, more experienced trainers. The older trainer teaches the younger one, who does most of the work. If the younger trainer is unable to complete a task or loses heart, the older trainer takes over.

Master trainers: teach, but also work with council leaders and the hierarchy. All members are required to come in from time to time for a "tune-up" (programming reinforcement), even senior leaders.

EEG machine: it is often equipped with abbreviated connections for quick use. It is widely used for brainwave programming; it also verifies that a certain alter is out when called. Can be used to verify deep trance state before beginning deep programming. Trainers learn to read this data.

Training table: a large table, often made of steel, covered with plastic or an easy-to-clean material. On the sides, at regular intervals, are arm, leg and neck restraints to prevent movement.

Trainer's chair: large chair with armrests. Restraints such as those described above will be placed at regular intervals to limit movement while the person is sitting in the chair.

Shock equipment: models and types vary widely, depending on age and company. Most have a set of rubber-coated wires, with electrodes that can be connected by Velcro, rubber (steel spikes pressed under finger and toe nails), or gel pads (larger areas of the body such as the chest, arms, legs). Some electrodes are tiny and can be stuck next to the eyes or placed in the genitals. These electrodes are connected to the "shock box", which has controls to determine the amount of electricity and frequency, if spaced shocks are desired.

Medications: a large number of opiates, barbiturates, hypnotics, sedatives, anesthetic agents. Resuscitation drugs and antidotes are also kept, clearly labeled and indexed. Many drugs, especially experimental drugs, are known only by code names, such as "alphin 1".

Cardiopulmonary resuscitation equipment: in case the person has an adverse reaction to the medication or programming. Occasionally, a child alter inadvertently exits during a programming sequence and is overdosed with medication intended for adult alters. The trainers must administer the antidote and resuscitate the child as if it were a real child. They are well aware of this fact and severely punish the alt children to teach them to go out only when called.

Virtual reality headsets: the keystone of recent years. Many programming sequences use holographic images and virtual reality devices, including assassination programs, where the person realistically "kills" another human being. These virtual drives are far more advanced than those in video game rooms.

Bodybuilding equipment: used in military training to improve physical condition and lean body mass.

Steel instruments: used to penetrate orifices and cause pain

Stretching machine: used as a punishment, it "stretches" the person without breaking the bones. Extremely painful.

Trainer's grids and projectors: used to project the grids onto the wall or ceiling.

Movie projector: to project movies, although new VR discs are replacing them. Computer: data collection and analysis; maintaining a computer grid on the person's system. Current military computer access codes will be used to download into government computers.

Trainer logs: contain indexed copies of the subject's systems, including key changes, command codes, etc.

Comforting objects: used to comfort the subject afterwards. This may be a toy or candy for the child alters, or oil for the massage. Hot towels or drinks may be offered as the trainer bonds with and comforts the person they have been working with. This is probably the most important part of the training process, as the trainer calmly and gently explains to the person that they did well and that they are proud of them.

FIRST CHAPTER

An overview of the Illuminati

To understand the programming of the Illuminati sect, it is necessary to first understand a little about the structure and philosophy of the organization. The Illuminati is a group of people who follow a philosophy known as "Illuminism" or "Enlightenment". The Illuminati were named several hundred years ago, but their roots and history can be traced back to the ancient mystery religions of Egypt, ancient Babylon and even Mesopotamia. From these ancient religions, practiced secretly for hundreds and hundreds of years, came esoteric groups that continued to practice the rituals, traditions and enculturation brought by the original groups.

Over the centuries, these groups have practiced openly in some countries, and secretly in countries where Christianity or other religions opposed their practices. Among the groups that emerged from these ancient roots were the Knights Templar, the Rosicrucians, Baptism, and the Druidic cults. These groups were the precursors, or roots, of modern Illuminism. Early Illuminist leaders chose to take what they felt were the best practices of each root religion, combine them into principles, and then organize those principles along specific guidelines.

Modern Enlightenment is a philosophy financed by the rich, but practiced in all social strata. It is a philosophy whose principles have spread throughout the world. It began with the German branch of the Rosicrucians, spread to England, and then arrived in the United States with the first settlers.

The Illuminati have three main branches: the Germanic branch, which oversees the others, the British branch, which handles finances, and the French/Russian branch. These three branches are represented in the United States and Canada, as well as in every country in the world.

How the Illuminati is organizing at United States

The Illuminati has groups in every major city in the United States.

They originally entered the U.S. through Pittsburgh, Pennsylvania, and from there they spread throughout the country. Eighteen U.S. cities are considered major "power centers" for Illuminati power and/or influence. These cities are Washington, DC and surrounding areas; Albany, New York; Pittsburgh, Pa. Winston Salem area "Golden Triangle"; Raleigh, NC; Minneapolis, Minn; Ann Arbor, Mich; Wichita, Kan; Phoenix, Az; Portland, Or; Flagstaff, Az; Seattle, Wash; Houston, TX; Los Angeles, CA and surrounding areas; Atlanta, Ga; New Orleans, La; Springfield, Miss. Other cities are also important to the Illuminati, but these cities provide them with money, conduct research and often house regional councils.

Hierarchy of the Illuminati

The Illuminati have organized their society into extremely hierarchical or stratified levels. In fact, the upper levels are known as the:

Hierarchical Level: The Illuminati have divided the United States into seven geographic regions. Each region has its own regional council, consisting of 13 members, with an advisory board of three elders for each. These regions interact in matters of finance, personnel, education, etc. Below each regional council is a local council. This is a 13-member council, the head of which sits on the regional council and provides input to the regional council on the local groups he leads. The local council also has an advisory board of 3 members.

A local governing board in a large metropolitan area might look like the following:

➢ Head of the local council (reports to the regional council)

➢ Two intermediaries (reporting to him/her on all activities under the responsibility of the lead partner)

➢ Four directors (oversee finances, administer, organize group activities)

➢ Six senior trainers (supervise trainers in local groups, train other trainers)

Below the aforementioned executive board are six individuals designated as informants or intermediaries, who attend local group meetings, interact with local group leaders, and report to the executive board.

Anarchic level: The levels below the governing board are called anarchic levels. Below the middle level is the local group level. It is made up of local "sister groups" (the number of which varies according to the size of the city or cities in the region). A large metropolitan area may have from ten to twenty-seven groups.

Each partner group will be led by: A High Priest and Priestess: this role rotates every three years to allow for different people within the group to take on leadership roles. Each group will also have different members with specific roles/work within the group. These roles will be discussed in Chapter 2.

One thing I'd like to point out is that the Illuminati today is generational. Their members were born into the group, which is highly organized, as described above. The organization described above is representative, with minor variations, of most major metropolitan areas in the United States. Smaller population centers will be organized along similar lines, but will be grouped with several cities in the region to create the local governing board.

How the Illuminati make money

The Illuminati are involved in many areas to make money, as they need continuous funding to survive. They are involved in many illegal as well as legal businesses.

➢ **Drug Trafficking:** The Illuminati partnered with the Mafia and the Colombians years ago to help each other bring drugs into the United States. They also provide couriers to get drugs and money out of the United States. Illuminists are usually wealthy businessmen who have four layers of people below them. The fourth layer is in contact with people in the drug industry. They never present themselves as illuminists, but only as people interested in investments, with a guaranteed profit, and are very discreet. In return, local groups provide people willing to serve as money or drug couriers, or people willing to help cover local operations.

➢ **Pornography:** In many cities, the Illuminati are linked to pornography, prostitution, child prostitution and the sale of white slaves. Again, there are several layers present, like a buffer, between the real "leadership" and those who participate in the activities, or fund them and end up getting paid for them.

➢ **Children:** are often provided by local cult groups and taught to become child prostitutes (and later adult prostitutes); they are photographed and filmed in all types of pornography available, including "snuff films" and violent films.

➢ **Arms trafficking:** The Illuminati and other groups are also involved in the international sale and shipment of arms. The Illuminati have well-trained couriers who cross international and national borders. These couriers are very discreet and do not reveal their sources, under penalty of suicide or assassination. These people are accountable to others above them, with two more "buffer layers" of people above them, before the Illuminati person with the money who is helping to fund all this is found.

➢ **Buying access codes to military computers:** The Illuminati will train people from all walks of life to meet near or on military bases. The typical person used may be an innocent-looking military wife, a local businessman, or even a student. A contact inside the base, also a dissociative illuminist, passes on information to the outside contact. Occasionally, the contact is paid in money, information or goods. Military computer codes are changed on a random schedule; the Illuminati have at least 5 or 6 contacts at each major base, who alert them when codes are about to be changed, on pain of death. The Illuminati like to have access to military computers because it gives them access to confidential files around the world.

➢ **Hiring and selling assassinations:** This practice exists all over the world, more in Europe than in the United States. These people are paid a lot of money to carry out a private or political assassination. The money is paid either to the assassin or to the trainer; usually the two share the fee. The assassin is given protection in another country for a period of time until the trail is cleared. If the assassination takes place in Europe, he may be sent to the Far East or the United States, and vice versa if the assassination takes place in the United States. The Illuminati have a wide range of locations and false identities to hide these people, unless for some reason they want to get rid of the assassin along with him. In this case, the assassin is captured and immediately executed.

➢ **Mercenaries/military trainers:** guess who gets paid to come and train paramilitary groups? Who has training camps in every state in Montana, Nevada and North Dakota? Who occasionally offers their expertise in exchange for a large financial reward? They never advertise themselves as Illuminati unless the group is known to be sympathetic to their cause. Instead, they are cold, brutal, hardcore military trainers who offer to teach these groups in exchange for money or, better yet, a promise of affiliation with their group (loyalty in exchange for knowledge). More and more paramilitary groups have been integrated into the Illuminati in this way, without them really knowing who and what the group is. This allows the Illuminati to monitor these groups (their trainers report on them and their activities), and it can be useful to have trained military groups that they can call upon one day.

➢ **Banking:** The early illuminists were bankers, and they have highly trained financiers to organize their money and channel the above illicit funds to more "respectable" front groups/organizations. They also create charities, community organizations, etc., which serve as fronts and receive money from large numbers of people. The Illuminati take particular pride in their money and manipulation skills, as well as their ability to expertly hide their paper trail layer by layer.

All the banking trails eventually lead to Belgium, the Illuminati financial center for the world. These are some of the major money-making ventures that the Illuminati are involved in. They have considerable financial resources to support their ventures, which means they can actually hire the best lawyers, accountants, etc. To help them cover their tracks.

CHAPTER TWO

Jobs in the Illuminati (or why they spend all their time training people)

To understand generational programming, one must understand WHY the cult goes to such lengths to introduce programming into people. Training is time and effort, and no one—especially a cult member—will spend that amount of energy if there is no return on investment. This is just an overview of some of the more common jobs in the cult. It is not an exhaustive or complete list.

The cult has a highly organized hierarchy of positions. Like any large organization, it needs people who are well trained in their jobs—so well trained that they can perform their tasks without even thinking about it—to function smoothly. To maintain secrecy, this group also needs people who are totally committed to not revealing their role in the cult, even under threat of death or punishment. The cult wants members who are totally loyal to the group and its principles, who never question the orders they are given. These qualities in group members guarantee the continuity of the cult and ensure that its secrets are never revealed to the outside world.

Here is a sample of some of the jobs in worship (not in order of priority)

➢ **Informers:** These people are trained to observe details and conversations with a photographic memory. They are trained to report to their local cult leader or hierarchy, or to their trainer, and will download large amounts of information under hypnotic trance. Detailed knowledge of conversations or even documents can often be retrieved in this manner. They are often used as "plants" to gather information in government circles and at cult meetings.

➢ **Breeders:** These people are often chosen from childhood to have and raise children. They may be chosen based on their lineage, or given in arranged marriages or cult alliances, to "breed" children. A parent will often sell the services of a child as a breeder to the local cult leader in exchange for favors or status. These children are rarely used as sacrifices; they are usually given to other cult members to adopt or raise, but the breeder is told that any child born to her has been "sacrificed" to prevent her from seeking the child. Sometimes, in anarchic cults, a local chief or relative has a child as a result of an incestuous affair. This child is given away or killed, but the mother is told that the child has been given to a distant branch and must be abandoned.

➢ **Prostitutes:** Prostitutes can be men or women of any age. They are trained from an early age to perform sexual favors for one or more adults in exchange for payment to the child's parents or the local cult group. Sometimes the prostitute may be given to a cult member on a temporary basis as a "reward" for a job well done. Child prostitution is an important activity for the cult, and the training of very young children for this role is taken very seriously. Child prostitutes are also used to blackmail political figures or leaders outside the sect.

➢ **Child pornography**: the child used in pornography (which can include bestiality) can also be of any age or gender. Child pornography is also a major commercial activity in cults, and includes snuff films. Children are trained in this role as early as preschool, often with the help or approval of their parents. Parents are paid or receive favors from the cult in exchange for selling their child or allowing them to train their child in this area.

➢ **Media personnel**: if they are very bright and verbal. They will be sent to journalism school and work for local or regional media outlets after graduation. These people have many contacts within the organization as well as in the outside world. They write books and articles favorable to the illuminist viewpoint without ever revealing their true affiliation. They tend to do biased research in their articles, favoring only one point of view, such as denying the existence of DID or ritual abuse. For example, they only interview psychiatrists/psychologists who favor that view and distort the data to present a convincing picture to the general public. If necessary, they will outright lie or invent data to support their view. Some group members have been deliberately trained to try to help form public opinion that cults do not exist (i.e., no rational person would believe this "mass hysteria"). Illuminists believe that to control the media is to control the thinking of the masses. This is why they take the training of media personnel very seriously. The cleaners meticulously clean up after the rituals. They walk the site after the ceremony, rake the area, etc. This work is taught to them as early as pre-school age.

➢ **Preparers: set up** tables, tablecloths, candles and other paraphernalia quickly and efficiently. This job is learned in childhood.

➢ **Readers:** They read from the Book of Illumination or from the archives of local groups; they also keep copies of sacred literature in a safe and are trained in ancient languages. Readers are valued for their clear voices and their ability to dramatize important passages and bring them to life.

➢ **Cutters:** They are taught to dissect animal or human sacrifices (they are also called the "slicers and cutters" of the sect). They can kill quickly, without emotion and efficiently. They are trained from an early age.

➢ **Chanters:** sing, sway or lead choirs of sacred songs on major sacred occasions.

➢ **High Priest/Priestess:** The person who holds this position changes every two years in most groups, although they may hold this position longer in smaller, more rural groups. These individuals administer and direct the local cult group, coordinate tasks within the cult, give assignments, and pass on meeting dates set by the local hierarchy or governing council. They also activate the local group's telephone tree, evaluate the performance of local group members and direct all spiritual activities. They report to the local or regional leadership council of their group.

➢ **Trainers:** These individuals teach local group members their assigned tasks and monitor the completion of those tasks at local group meetings or after an assigned task. They report to the high priest/priestess of their group, as well as to the local lead trainer of the Leadership Council.

➢ **Punishers:** These are the people who brutally punish or discipline members caught breaking the rules or acting outside or above their authority. They are universally despised by other cult members, even if the local high priest or priestess will praise them for a job well done. Usually physically strong, they will use whatever methods are deemed necessary to prevent the undesirable behavior from recurring. Punishment may be public or private, depending on the severity of the offense. Each local group has several punishers.

➤ **Trackers:** These individuals track and monitor members who attempt to leave their local group. They are trained to use dogs, firearms, tasers, and all necessary tracking techniques. They also know how to use the Internet to monitor a person's activities. They track credit card usage, checks written, and other methods to find a missing person.

➤ **Teachers:** These people give group classes to children to teach them philosophy, languages and specialized areas of the cult.

➤ **Childcare:** These individuals care for very young children when the adults are at the local group meeting. Generally, care is provided only for young children. After the age of two, the children regularly participate in a group activity led by the trainers of the younger children. The child care workers are generally calm and coolly efficient.

➤ **Smugglers:** These members smuggle weapons, money, drugs or illegal items from one state or country to another. They are usually young, single people who are not accountable to the outside world. They are trained to use firearms to get out of difficult situations. They must be reliable and able to overcome all expected obstacles.

➤ **Commanders:** These individuals oversee military training in local groups and assist in the successful conduct of these exercises. They delegate tasks to their subordinates and are responsible to the local leadership council. The board has at least one member representing the military branch of the Illuminati. In addition, there are many military-related positions under the commanders.

➤ **Behavioral scientists:** These individuals often oversee training in local and regional groups. These students of human behavior are intensely involved in data collection and human experimentation in the name of furthering the knowledge of human behavior in the scientific field. They are almost always cold, methodical, impersonal people who will employ any method to study trauma and its effects on human personality.

Their main interest is to implement cult programming and control in the most effective and long-lasting way possible.

There are many other jobs within the cult. The cult spends much of its time getting people to do these jobs for it for FREE, so it PROGRAMS people to believe they are doing their "family" and the world a favor. The reality, of course, is that the person is being abused and exploited by the cult.

CHAPTER THREE

Second conspiracy theory, or the Illuminati plan for world domination (known as "Novus Ordem Seclorum")

B efore discussing the actual programming techniques, it is important to understand the philosophy behind why the Illuminists program people. All groups have goals, and the Illuminati are no exception. Money is not their end goal, it is a means to an end. That end, or goal, is nothing less than to rule the world. The Illuminati have a fixed plan, similar to the Soviet Union's "five-year" and "ten-year" plans. This is what the Illuminati themselves believe and teach their followers as gospel truth.

Whether they will succeed is another matter entirely. This is the Illuminati agenda on ALL levels. As with any goal, the Illuminati have specific steps they plan to implement to achieve their goals. In short, each region of the United States has "nerve centers" or power bases for regional activity. The United States has been divided into seven major geographic regions. Each region includes locations of military complexes and bases hidden in remote and isolated areas or on large private properties.

These bases are used intermittently to teach and train generations of Illuminati in military techniques, unarmed combat, crowd control, weapons handling and all aspects of military warfare. Why? Because the Illuminati believe that our government, as we know it, and the governments of most of the nations of the world, are destined to collapse. These will be planned collapses, which will occur in the following manner:

The Illuminati first planned a financial collapse that will make the Great Depression look like a picnic. This will happen through the maneuvering of the world's major banks and financial institutions, stock manipulation and interest rate changes. Most people will be in debt to the federal government through bank debt, credit cards, etc. The governments will immediately recall all debts, but most people will be unable to pay and will be ruined. This will cause a widespread financial panic that will occur simultaneously around the world, as the Illuminati believe strongly in controlling people through finances.

Then there will be a military takeover, region by region, when the government declares a state of emergency and martial law. People will have panicked, there will be a state of anarchy in most localities, and the government will justify its action as necessary to control the panicked citizens. The cult-trained military leaders and the people under their direction will use weapons and crowd control techniques to implement this new state of affairs. This is why so many survivors under the age of 36 report having gone through a military program. People who are not illuminists or sympathetic to their cause will resist. The Illuminists expect this and will (and are) trained to deal with it. They train their people in hand-to-hand combat, crowd control and, if necessary, will kill to control the crowds. The Illuminati train their members to be prepared for every possible reaction to the takeover. Many victims of mind control will also be called to work with pre-set command codes. These codes are intended to summon a new system of presentation, entirely faithful to the cult. Trauma-programmed destruction codes will be used to destroy or bury alters who are not loyal to the cult.

Military bases will be set up in every community (in fact, they already exist, but are secret). In the next few years, they will be built and revealed. Each community will have regional bases and leaders to whom they will be accountable. The hierarchy will closely mirror the current secret hierarchy.

About five years ago, when I left the Illuminati, about 1% of the U.S. population was either part of the Illuminati, supportive of the Illuminati, or a victim of Mind Control (and therefore considered usable).

This may not seem like much, but imagine 1% of the population highly trained in the use of weapons, crowd control, psychological and behavioral techniques, armed with weapons and linked to paramilitary groups.

These people will also be completely dedicated to their cause. The Illuminati firmly believe that they can easily defeat the remaining 99% of the population, most of whom are untrained, or poorly trained, as "weekend hunters." Even the local army will be defeated, because the Illuminati will have regional cells with highly trained leaders. They are also counting on the element of surprise to take power. Many of the top leaders of the Illuminati's militia wing are or have been officers in the military, and thus already have a good knowledge of the most effective techniques for overcoming the defenses of a region or locality.

After the military takeover, the population will have the option of embracing the Illuminati cause or rejecting it (with imprisonment, suffering, and even death as possible punishments). These people firmly believe that the intelligent, the "enlightened" or the Illuminati are born to rule. They are arrogant and view the general population as "stupid sheep" who will be easily led if offered strong leadership, financial assistance in an unstable world economy, and disastrous consequences if the person rebels. Their ruthlessness and ability to implement their agenda should not be minimized.

Illuminati banking leaders such as the Rothschilds, Vanderbilts, Rockefellers, Carnegies and Mellons, for example, will come forward and propose to "save" the ailing world economy. A new monetary exchange system, based on an international monetary system and based between Cairo, Egypt, and Brussels, Belgium, will be established. A true "One World Economy", creating the long awaited "One World Order", will become a reality.

The Illuminati agenda does not end there, but this is the core of it. This agenda is what the Illuminati really, truly believe in, teach and train for. They are willing to sacrifice their lives for this cause, to teach the next generation, because they believe their children are their legacy. I was told that my children's generation would see this empowerment in the 21st century. At this time, the Illuminati have quietly and secretly furthered their takeover plan through their infiltration goals:

1. The media

2. The banking system

3. The educational system

4. Government, both local and federal

5. The scientific world

6. The churches

They are working now, and have been for several hundred years, to take over these six areas. They do NOT show up at an institution and say, "Hi, I'm a local illuminist and I'd like to take over your bank.") Instead, they begin by having several people quietly invest funds over several years, gradually buying more and more shares of the bank (or other institution they wish to control), until they have financial control. They never openly disclose their agenda or cultic activities, as they often have amnesia. They are highly respected, "Christian" looking business leaders within the community. Image in the community is very important to an Illuminist; they will do anything to maintain a normal and respected facade, and DESPERATE to be exposed. In one leadership of a large metropolitan city, of which I was a member, sat: a head of the local small business administration; a CEO of a government defense contractor; a principal of a Christian school; a deputy mayor of the city; a journalist; a nurse; a doctor; a behavioral psychologist; an Army colonel; and a Navy commander. All but one attended church weekly; all were highly respected in the community.

NONE of them appeared "evil" or "nasty".

If you met them in person, you would probably instantly like either of these smart, communicative, friendly, even charismatic people. This is their biggest cover, as we often expect great evil to "appear" as such, as portrayed in the media as causing changes in people's faces and behavior, or marking them like the biblical Cain. None of the illuminists I have known were evil or looked evil in their everyday lives, although some were dysfunctional, like alcoholics. The dissociation that animates the illuminists is their best cover for going undetected at this time. Many, if not most, of these people are completely unaware of the great evil they are involved in overnight.

There are other groups that are not part of the Illuminati, but the Illuminati know about them. The Illuminati are not the only group that follows esoteric practices or worships ancient deities or demons. They encourage division between different groups (divide and conquer is one of their guiding principles) and do not care about other groups. Instead, they often welcome them under their umbrella, if possible. This has been happening more and more in recent years as the Illuminati teach their training principles, which are considered the best by most secret groups, in exchange for loyalty to the Illuminati. They send their trainers to these groups, and these trainers report to the local regional council.

In the political arena, the Illuminati will fund both sides of a race, for their greatest maxim is that "out of chaos comes order," or the discipline of anarchy. That is why they have sent weapons and funded both sides of the two great world wars of this century. They believe that history is a game, like chess, and that only through strategy, combat, conflict and testing can the strongest emerge. I no longer agree with this philosophy, but at one time I did, wholeheartedly. Hopefully, as these people and their agenda are revealed, the man in the street will rise up against this rule intended to be imposed on unsuspecting humanity.

CHAPTER FOUR

How the Illuminati programs people: an overview of some basic types of programming

In the first few chapters, I defined Illuminism, its scope, and some of the philosophies, money-making ventures, and programs that help explain WHY they program people. I think it's important to understand these things, as a preface to the following chapters. Why? The programming techniques I will describe require an incredible amount of effort, time, dedication and planning on the part of the cult to apply to the individual. Only a group of highly motivated people would devote the time to this task. These chapters are very difficult for me, as an individual, to write since my role in the cult was that of a programmer. Thus, the techniques you are about to read about were often those I used to program the people I worked with. The reason I am writing this book is because I believe that therapists who work with DID, as well as survivors, deserve to know WHAT is being done to people, HOW it is being done, and to be given some ideas on how to undo the programming that the cult places in people.

First, I would like to address the issue of unintentional versus intentional programming. This is called the environmental milieu in which the child is raised. The programming of an Illuminati generational child often begins before birth (more on this later), but once born, the very environment in which the child is raised becomes a form of programming. Often the infant is raised in a home environment that combines daytime abandonment and dysfunctional parental figures. The infant quickly learns that nighttime and worship activities are most important. He or she may be deprived of attention, even abused, during the day, and is treated as special or "seen" by parents only within the cult setting. This can lead to very young alters around the core or splits in the core, who feel "invisible," abandoned, rejected, unworthy of love or attention, or who think they don't even exist unless they are doing work for their "family."

Another conditioning environment and process that the infant must face is the fact that the adults around him/her are INCONSISTENT, since the adults in a generational cult family are almost always also multiple or DID. For the infant, this means that the parents act one way at home, a totally different way at cult meetings, and an even different way in normal society.

Because these are the infant's first experiences with adults and their behaviors, he or she has no choice but to accept the reality that human beings act in strikingly different ways in different contexts. Although involuntary, this behavior prepares the infant for later dissociation through mimicry with the adults around him.

Intentional programming

The intentional programming of a child by the Illuminati often begins before birth. Prenatal splitting is well known in the cult, as the fetus is quite capable of splitting in the womb as a result of trauma. This operation usually takes place between the seventh and ninth month of pregnancy. The techniques used involve placing headphones on the mother's abdomen and playing loud, discordant music (such as certain modern classical pieces or even Wagner operas). Heavy, loud rock music has also been used. Other methods include having the mother ingest quantities of bitter substances, to make the amniotic fluid bitter, or yelling at the fetus inside the womb. The mother's abdomen may also be hit. Mild shocks to the abdomen may be applied, especially when the term is near, and may be used to induce premature labor or to ensure that the child is born at a ceremonial celebration. Some labor-inducing drugs may also be administered if a certain birth date is desired.

Once the child is born, testing begins very early, usually in the first few weeks of life. The trainers, who have been taught to look for certain qualities in the infant, place it on a table, on a velvet cloth, and test its reflexes to various stimuli. The infant's strength, reaction to heat, cold and pain are tested. Each child reacts differently and the trainers look for dissociation, quick reflexes and reaction times. They also encourage early dissociation in the infant through these tests.

The infant will also be abused, in order to create fragments. Methods of abuse may include: rectal probes, digital anal rape, low-level electric shocks to fingers, toes and genitals, cutting of genitals as part of a ritual (in older infants). The goal is to begin fragmentation before a true ego state develops and to accustom the infant to pain and reflexive dissociation from pain (yes, even very small infants dissociate; I have seen it many times; they light up with a soft white or glassy light in the face of continued trauma).

Isolation and abandonment programs are sometimes implemented in a rudimentary manner. The infant is abandoned or not cared for by adults, intentionally during the day, and then picked up, soothed, cleaned, and cared for in preparation for a ritual or group gathering. This is to help the infant associate nighttime gatherings with "love" and care, and to help the process of attachment to the cult or "family". The infant will learn to associate maternal attention with participation in rituals and will eventually associate cult gatherings with a sense of security.

As the child grows older, between 15 and 18 months, the child is further fragmented by having parents and cult members abuse the child in a more methodical manner. This is done by intermittently soothing the infant, bonding with it, and then shocking it on the fingers; the infant may be dropped from a height onto a rug or mattress and taunted as it lies scared and terrified, crying. He may be placed in cages for a period of time or exposed to short periods of isolation. Deprivation of food, water and basic needs may begin later in this phase. All of these methods are intended to create intentional dissociation in the infant. The infant at this age may be taken to group meetings, but other than special occasions or dedications, will not yet have an active role in the cult setting. Small children are usually assigned to a cult member, or janitor, to watch over them during group activities; this janitor role is usually rotated among lower-level members or teenagers.

Between 20 and 24 months, the toddler can begin to follow the "steps of discipline" that the Illuminati use to teach their children. The age at which the child begins them varies depending on the group, the parent, the trainer and the child. These "stages of discipline" should be called "stages of torment and abuse" because their goal is to create a very dissociated, emotionally disconnected child who is completely and unconsciously loyal to the cult. The order of the stages can also be changed slightly, depending on the whims of the trainer or the parents.

I will first discuss the first five steps of the discipline: (note: these steps may vary somewhat from region to region, but most follow at least roughly this pattern, even if not in the same order).

First step: don't need

The young child is placed in a room devoid of sensory stimuli, usually a training room with gray, white or beige walls. The adult leaves and the child is left alone for periods of time that can vary from a few hours to a full day as the child grows. If the child begs the adult to stay and not leave, or screams, the child is beaten and told that the periods of isolation will increase until the child learns to stop being weak. The apparent purpose of this discipline is to teach the child to rely on his or her own internal resources, not on outsiders ("reinforcing"). What it actually does is create in the child a tremendous terror of abandonment. When the adult, or trainer, returns to the room, the child cradles or huddles in a corner, sometimes almost catatonic with fear. The trainer will then "rescue" the child, feed them, give them something to drink, and bond with them as a "rescuer." The puppy trainer will tell them that the "family" has asked the puppy trainer to save the child because the family "loves" the child.

The trainer will instill the teachings of the cult, at this point, in the helpless, fearful and almost insanely grateful child who has just been "saved" from isolation. The trainer will repeatedly tell the child how much he or she needs the family that has just saved him or her from death by starvation or abandonment. The very young child will learn to associate comfort and security with the attachment to the trainer, who may be a parent, and the presence of "family" members. The cult is very familiar with the principles of child development and has developed exercises such as those described above after hundreds of years of teaching very young children.

Second step: don't want to

This stage is very similar to the first stage and actually reinforces it. It will be done intermittently with the first stage over the next few years of the child's life. Once again, the child is left alone in a training room or isolated room without food or water for an extended period of time. An adult enters the room with a large pitcher of ice water or food. If the child asks for either, while the adult eats or drinks in front of him, he is severely punished for being weak and needy. This stage is reinforced until the child learns not to ask for food or water unless it is offered first. The ostensible reason given by the cult for this stage is that it creates a strong child who can go without food and water for longer and longer periods of time. The real reason is that it creates a child who is completely dissociated from his or her own needs for food, water, or other comforts, who is afraid to ask outside adults for help. This creates a hyper-vigilance in the child, as he learns to seek out outside adults to know when he can meet his needs, and not to trust his own body's signals. The child is already learning to look to others to tell him how he should think or feel, instead of relying on his own feelings. The cult then becomes the child's place of control.

Step three: Don't want to

The child is placed in a room with his/her favorite toys or objects. A caring adult enters the room and plays with the child. This adult can be a friend, aunt, parent or trainer. The child and adult can play fantasy games about the child's wishes, dreams or secret desires. This happens repeatedly, and the child's trust is slowly earned. Thereafter, the child is severely punished for any aspect of his or her wishes or fantasies shared with the adult, including destroying favorite toys, going to undo or destroy secret places of safety the child may have created, or even destroying non-cult protectors. This stage is repeated, with variations, many times over the next few years. Sometimes the child's siblings, parents, or friends are used to reveal inner fantasies that the child has revealed to them during the day or in unsupervised moments. The ostensible reason given by the cult for this step is to create a child who does not fantasize, who is more outward looking and less inward looking. In other words, the child must look to adults for permission in all aspects of his or her life, including the inside. In reality, this stage destroys all the safe places the child has created internally to retreat from the horrors he or she is experiencing. This step creates a sense in the child that there is no real safety, that the cult will find out everything they think. Exercises like this are also used to create young alters in the child who will themselves point out to the cult trainers the secret places of safety or hidden wishes against the cult that other alters have. This then begins to create a hostility and division between the systems, which the cult will manipulate throughout the person's life in order to control them.

Fourth stage: survival of the fittest

This stage begins to create alter-aggressors in the young child. ALL MEMBERS OF THE CULT ARE CALLED UPON TO BECOME AGGRESSORS; THIS BEGINS IN EARLY CHILDHOOD.

The child is brought into a room with a trainer and another child of the same age, or slightly younger, than the child being taught. The child is beaten severely, for a long period of time, by the trainer, and then asked to hit the other child in the room or he will be beaten again. If the child refuses, he or she is severely punished, the other child is also punished, and then the child is asked to punish the other child. If the child continues to refuse, cry, or try to hit the trainer instead, he or she will continue to be beaten severely and will be told to hit the other child, in order to direct his or her anger at the other child. This stage is repeated until the child complies. This stage begins around the age of two or two and a half and is used to create aggressive changes in the young child. As the child gets older, the punishments become more and more brutal. Children are expected to become aggressors of others at a very young age and to practice on children younger than themselves, with the encouragement and rewards of the adults around them. They also mimic these adults, who consistently view perpetration as normal. The child will learn that this is an acceptable outlet for their aggressive impulses and rage generated by the brutality to which they are constantly exposed.

Fifth step: the code of silence

There are many, many schemes used to set this up, starting at about age two, when the child begins to become more verbal. Usually, after a ritual or group meeting, the child is asked about what he or she saw or heard during the meeting. Like most obedient young children, they comply. They are immediately severely beaten or tortured, and a new alter is created, who is asked to keep the memories of what he or she saw, or risk losing his or her life. The new part always agrees. The child and this new party are subjected to a ceremony in which they swear never to tell, and alters are created whose role is to kill the body if the other parties remember.

The child is also subjected to severe psychological torture to ensure that he or she will never be tempted to talk, including: being buried alive; being almost drowned; witnessing "treacherous deaths" involving slow painful tortures, such as being burned or flayed alive; being buried with a partially rotten corpse and being told that he or she will become a corpse like him or her if he or she ever talks, etc. The scenarios follow one another, invented by people with infinitely cruel imaginations, in order to guarantee the secrecy of the young child. These methods have been perfected over hundreds of years of the cult's practice with its children. The reason these things are done is obvious: the cult is involved in criminal activities, as explained in the early chapters of this book, and it wants to ensure the continued silence of its children. This is one of the reasons why the cult has survived so long and, along with its veil of secrecy, why more and more survivors are afraid or unwilling to reveal the abuse they have suffered. To reveal the secrets of the cult, a child must face some of the most horrific psychological trauma and abuse imaginable; even as an adult, the survivor finds it difficult to put these things aside when talking about the abuse he or she has suffered. Children and adults alike are told that if they speak out, they will be hunted down and shot (assassin training lets the child know that this is not an idle threat), that they will be slowly tortured. Throughout childhood, the child is exposed to dramatizations and role-playing that reinforce this.

Suggestions that can help

I believe in offering ideas on how to undo some of the programs mentioned above as well, because I don't believe in knowledge just for the sake of knowledge. The survivor often needs tools to try to undo some of the horrific abuse that the cult put them through, especially when memories of these things come back to them. THESE ARE SIMPLY HELPFUL TIPS AND ARE NOT A SUBSTITUTE FOR THE ADVICE OF A GOOD THERAPIST.

1. Early Childhood Programming:

This is difficult to address because it touches on fundamental issues of abandonment and rejection for the survivor. These are often the very first experiences the survivor had as a child in relationships with parents and key family members. Working on this requires the whole-hearted effort of all the alter-systems within, to join in the nurturing of the divisive core that experienced severe parental rejection, and the cognitive recognition that the DAY was also important; that the adults around the child were the ones who were unhealthy. Infants often feel unlovable, overly needy, depressed; but inner alters can comfort them and share the reality that the infant was truly lovable, regardless of the behavior of the outer adults around them. Again, a supportive outside therapist and a strong, nurturing belief system can help tremendously in the healing process, as new messages are brought to the abandoned and wounded parts. It will take time to sort out what has happened, to grieve the real abandonment issues and to bring reality to very young and deeply wounded parts.

2. Early intentional fragmentation: (0–24 months)

Usually there are cognitive parts of the survivor inside, who have never forgotten the abuse, and who can help share the cognitive reality of the abuse with the amnesic alters. This needs to happen very slowly, given that the first abuse occurred very early in life. Creating an internal child's room, with safe toys and objects, can help. Older adults in the room can help hold and care for injured children in the room, while acknowledging and grieving the abuse that occurred. It is important to believe and validate the young parties when they come forward to share. It may be helpful to allow them to express themselves non-verbally, as these are very young children who often cannot yet speak. Having older children, close to the infants, verbalize their wants, needs, and fears can also help, as younger children often do not trust ANY adults, even those on the inside. A strong, caring outside therapist is also important for healing, modeling healthy parenting to a system that may have no idea, while balancing the child's need to be nurtured from the outside with the need for the internal system(s) to learn their own self-education skills. Internal helpers can reach out to the infants, anchor them, share the present reality (the body is older, the infants are safe, etc.), and help them to learn the skills they need. These helpers may be older internal children, as mentioned earlier). The survivor may also want to find supportive adults, whenever possible, who can help model healthy caregiving with good boundaries.

A THERAPIST OR FRIEND CANNOT RAISE THE SURVIVOR AGAIN. The survivor will want to, but in reality, he or she has had only one set of parents, good or bad, even sadly terrible. No outside person can come in and re-parent another person completely. What the therapist and support person can offer is caring, empathy, and listening while the survivor grieves the loss of a proper upbringing. They can offer friendship or empathy with good boundaries. They cannot become the survivor's parents, or the therapy will not progress. Instead, the entanglement will begin.

3. **The first five steps of the discipline (there are twelve in total; others will be covered in later chapters)**

Try to find the parts that have been abused. This may involve mapping the system (drawing pictures of what things look like on the inside) and reaching out to the cognizers (intellectuals) or controllers (business leaders on the inside) for information. An internal helper, or recorder, can also be extremely useful for this purpose.

Allow these parts to slowly acknowledge the agony they experienced during their deprivation: heat (being held over a fire or stove), cold (being placed in a freezer or ice, for example), lack of food, etc. Encourage sharing of the cognitive part of the memories first, while allowing the amnesic alters to grieve by "hearing about" these things. Allow them time to absorb these traumas, as they occurred over several years in early childhood, and will take time to process.

Healing cannot be rushed. Allow the alters to come forward later and share their feelings, while the more cognitive or helping parts are inside holding their hand, anchoring them in the here and now throughout the remembering process. Be prepared for floods of emotions at times, as well as bodily memories, when the abuse is recalled. A group of people on the inside can be designated as a "grounding team" to help ground these parts as they step forward and share their memories.

Safe remembering requires that the person has a trained therapist and has laid the foundation for good cooperation within the system, as discussed above. Memory work should not be done until there is good communication and cooperation within the system, otherwise the person will be overwhelmed by the memories as they come up. He or she will be overwhelmed and re-traumatized instead of helped, and may decompensate.

With good communication, memories can be evoked bit by bit, in manageable chunks, while cognitive alters continually help the survivor not to sink completely into the memory, and they can also help to root out the most injured parts.

The cult subjects people to certain types of programs in order to achieve a specific goal: to separate a person's intellect, or cognition, from their feelings. In these systems, cognitive alters are always considered "higher" than feeling alters; cognitive alters are taught to "pass on" their feelings to "lower" feeling alters. Although these labels are false, the cognitive alters will be afraid to feel the intense and overwhelming emotions that have caused them to separate more and more from the limbic alters, or sentient alters, within the system. This will have the effect of keeping the system divided in the survivor. It is important for the cognitive alters to realize that the sensory alters are part of them; that they can practice sharing their feelings in SMALL steps without needing to be inundated or overwhelmed.

A reminder: EXTERNAL SECURITY IS PRIMARY TO VOIDING INTERNAL PROGRAMMING.

You MUST be able to promise these parties external security and keep that promise, or they will understandably be reluctant to work internally to undo the programming. Why would they try to change, only to go back and be punished again? No system will undo its own protective dissociation if the abuse is permanent, otherwise it will continue to destabilize and dissociate again and again. Indeed, to dismantle dissociation would be to dismantle its own survival and protection. Stopping contact with the abusers and getting a safe therapist are the very first steps to take before trying to undo the internal programming. A system can still work on stopping contact with cults and begin to heal, while being accessible, but this will slow down therapy considerably, as the internal energy will be diverted to staying safe rather than repairing the trauma. A person can heal, and most survivors are still in contact with a cult when they begin therapy. BUT progress will be much faster once contact with the cult is broken (see chapter on preventing access to the survivor).

CHAPTER FIVE

Colors, metals and jewelry programming

One form of programming that is quite common among the Illuminati is color programming. Why is this done? The answer is that trainers are human beings and they are quite lazy. Color coding is a simple way to organize systems and allows the trainer to easily call up alters within a system. With the thousands of fragments that many multiples have in the cult, colors are a way to organize them into an easily accessible group.

In addition, young children recognize colors before they can read, so this training can take place quite early. In most children, it begins around the age of two.

How does it happen? The child is taken to a room with white, beige or colored walls. If the room is a neutral color, the lights in the room will be changed so that the room is colored with the color of the light. If blue is the color that is printed, the trainer will call a young child alter, either a controller or the core of a system. He or she will tell the child that he or she is going to learn how to become blue and what blue means. The room is bathed in blue light, as shown, or has been painted blue for use in this type of programming. The trainer is dressed in blue and may even wear a blue mask. Blue objects are placed around the room. The alter inside the child is called, drugged, hypnotized and traumatized on the table. As he wakes up from the trauma, still in a trance, he is told that blue is good and that he is blue. That blue is important. That blue will protect them from harm. That blue people are not harmed. This will go on for a while.

They then ask the child if they want to be "blue" like the trainers. If the child says yes, they continue. If the child says no, they will be traumatized again until they say yes. The child is often naked and told that they cannot wear clothes until they have "earned" the right to wear nice blue clothes. The "safety of being blue" (i.e., the absence of danger) and the danger of not having color are constantly emphasized. After a while, children really want to be blue. You can give them blue candy to reward them for choosing that color. You can give them blue sunglasses or tinted glasses.

They are allowed to wear blue dresses as long as they identify with the color chosen for them.

Once the child fully identifies with the color (or rather, the main alter or model in the system accepts that color), they are taught in incremental steps, over many training sessions, what the color blue means. They participate in dramas with other blue children, where they play the role of a "blue". They are drugged, hypnotized, traumatized, while the meaning of blue is instilled in them again and again. They are forced to act "blue". Depending on the trainer and the region, the meaning of the different colors varies. Many military systems are blue coded, or protective. Military alters are all called in periodically to reinforce the blue formation. If, at a later date, the trainer wants to access a blue system, they can call them by color, or wear a garment or scarf of the color they want to reach.

This becomes an unconscious trigger for that color to manifest itself. Color coding is one of the earliest methods used in systems. An entire system can be color coded with one color, or two or more colors, with each system controller (most systems have three) receiving a different color for its part of the system.

Metal programming

Metal programming is a type of programming that many children receive from the Illuminati. Since it is very similar to jewelry programming, I will talk about how it plays out in jewelry. Metals can range from bronze (the lowest) to platinum (the highest).

Jewelry programming

Many Illuminati children are subjected to either metal or jewelry programming, and sometimes both. Jewelry is considered higher than metals and more difficult to obtain. Which program is chosen and when it is applied depends on the status of the child, the status of his parents, the area in which he was born, the group into which he was born, and the trainers who work with him.

Basically, metals or jewelry are a form of reward-based programming. Here's how it works:

The child is shown a piece of jewelry such as a ring, or a large example of the jewelry (or metal) that is being put on. The child is asked, "Isn't this amethyst, this ruby, this emerald, this diamond beautiful? The child will be eager to look at it, to touch it, and will be encouraged to do so by a soft-spoken trainer. The trainer will ask the child, "Wouldn't you like to be as beautiful as this jewel (or metal jewel)?" The child is usually enthusiastic. Here is a sparkling gem, placed in his little hands (training often starts between two and three years old). Of course, he wants to be beautiful, sparkling, valued. The trainer will extol the beauty of the gemstone (or metal), tell the child how special, precious and sought after gems are, and essentially develop the idea of becoming like a jewel.

He is then told that in order to become a jewel, he must "earn the right". This involves

A.) Passing through the stages of discipline (see Chapter 3)

B.) Successful completion of "special tests

C.) Be recognized for a particular achievement

Becoming a jewel (or a precious metal) is presented to the little child as a carrot for doing well in training sessions. Obtaining a jewel is linked to moving up the ladder in the long and arduous training process expected of Illuminati children; having a jewel or metal means moving up and being praised. But the price is enduring hours of abuse called "training" but which is really organized and systemic abuse aimed at making the child what the trainer wants them to become.

Over time, with the help of drugs, hypnosis, shocks and other traumas, as the child goes through its formative process, it will begin to gain its jewels and/or metals, one by one. These will become full-fledged alters within.

Amethyst is usually the first to be earned, and is related to keeping secrets, never talking about them, and passing the first stage of discipline. Each stage is related to receiving a piece of jewelry or a precious metal.

The ruby will often be next, and it is linked to sexual abuse and sexual alters within. When the child is repeatedly sexually traumatized and survives, or creates sexual alterations to please the adults, they are "rewarded" by being allowed to become a ruby.

Emerald often comes later (between 12 and 15 years old). It is considered very valuable and is linked to family loyalty, witchcraft and spiritual fulfillment. Emeralds are often associated with a black cat or "familiar".

The diamond is the highest gemstone and not all children will obtain it. It is considered a great achievement and can only be obtained in adulthood, after passing rigorous tests. It is the control stone of a gemstone system. A diamond has passed the twelve stages of discipline, passed unusual tests and shown the greatest loyalty to his family.

The "family jewels" are often passed down internally during training sessions with trainers and family members. All major Illuminati families have jewels hidden in secret vaults (real jewels) that are passed down from generation to generation.

Children are often given a piece of jewelry to wear during the day as a reminder or reward once they have successfully completed their programming. A child may receive a ruby ring or garnet pin to wear; in fact, a grandparent or parent may insist that the child wear it. On ritual occasions, the child will be allowed to wear jewelry from the family vault, once he or she reaches a certain status. He may be allowed to wear a ruby pendant or an emerald bracelet at important rituals, and he will be very proud of it, for the sect is first and foremost, and always, an extremely status-conscious group. The children realize this and the adults make a big deal of the children earning the right to wear jewelry. This gives them a strong incentive to earn it.

Suggestions to help implement these forms of programming:

Color Programming: It is important to have good internal communication with internal alters and an external therapist during color programming work. If an individual finds that certain parts of their body believe they are a certain color, or if this is brought up in therapy, they will want to find out if possible how they came to have this belief system. Slowly discovering how the colors were introduced can help. Grieving for the large amount of deception, the amount of abuse inflicted on the child, and the very young alters who were the original models can occur. These parties may be barely verbal and want to draw their experiences, or use colors in collages (with the help of the older parties inside), to describe to a safe outsider what their reality has been. It can be helpful to let them know that they are NOT just a color and that they are part of a whole person. For a time, the survivor may see colored overlays as they are undoing this programming, and the inner parts share their memories. This is normal, although it may be unpleasant to see objects in yellow or green, for example. Grounding, cognitive reality orientation and patience will help the survivor through this period.

The programming of jewelry and metals can be more complex, as the child's sense of specialness, pride and status can be tied to these alters. Rubies, emeralds and diamonds are considered "high alters" internally and are used for leadership roles, both internally and externally. Recognizing their importance to the system, listening to them mourn their departure from the cult, which means giving up their status on the outside, and giving them new positions on the inside that are important can help. They can become leaders in the system by helping the person stay safe, once they have made the decision to leave the cult, and become strong allies. But they will often be among the most resistant, even hostile, to the idea of leaving the cult at first, because they have only known and remembered being rewarded for a job well done, and have learned to "pass on" trauma to the "lower parts" within the cult. They often do not sincerely believe that they were mistreated and only remember being petted or allowed to lead, or being told that they were special, that they were valuable.

It is helpful to listen to how they feel, recognize that leaving involves giving up things that were important to them, find out what their needs are, and try to find healthy ways to meet their needs outside of cult meetings. Allowing a gem to have leadership inside or chair internal meetings can compensate for the loss of external leadership when the survivor leaves the cult.

It is also important to recognize their importance to the survivor. Recognize that these parts are EXTREMELY disassociated from their own abuse/trauma and are in no rush to remember. But the survivor and a good therapist can gently bring them back to reality by letting them know that they were abused, that they are in fact part of the "lower emotional parts" that were abused, and that they will eventually have to acknowledge this. This takes time and good outside support. Allow them to express their feelings. They will often be very cognitive at first, but the feelings will come, especially the grief, then the pain of having been deceived by the cult, then the anguish of realizing that the abuse they passed on to others inside was actually happening to them. They may become very depressed at this stage, but they will also bring considerable stability and strength to the system, remaining safe and cult-free, once they reach this stage.

Here are some thoughts on programming colors, metals and jewelry. Other types of programming will be discussed in the next chapter.

CHAPTER SIX

Brain wave programming

In this chapter, I will discuss brainwave programming. Brainwave programming, like any other programming, depends on several factors. These include the child's ability to disassociate, the region of the country or country in which the child is growing up, the skill level of the trainers with whom the child is in contact, the physical resources and equipment available. There is no single "recipe" that works for every person and it would be ridiculous to say that everyone who undergoes brainwave programming does so in the same way. More and more programmers are talking to each other, sharing their knowledge on the net, both nationally and internationally, and exchanging their successes and failures. But there is no standardized methodology for brainwave programming. It is often influenced by the child himself, as well as by the whims of the trainer. Different groups may organize the systems differently or try to achieve different effects.

That said, what is brainwave programming? In simple terms, brainwave programming is when a young child enters a deep trance state, where they then learn to dissociate into a certain brainwave pattern. This is a complex skill, and not all children can do it. The goal is for the child to reach, for example, a coherent delta state, where delta brain waves appear on the eeg, which is attached to the child's head by electrodes in the scalp. Typically, two or even three trainers work with a child during the initial phases. One of them will "prepare" the child by using a hypnotic drug to induce a trance-like state. They will also have placed electrodes on the head, using a shortened version of the method used in a traditional hospital setting. If the delta state is induced, only the electrodes needed to pick up delta waves will be placed, for example. This saves time.

The prepared child will be placed on a "practice table" and will be very relaxed. The average child is about eight years old when this practice is started, as the cerebral cortex and neurological development are not sufficiently advanced at earlier ages (this practice has been tried at earlier ages, without much success, in the past; it was abandoned because of the neurological damage and "inability to pace" that the trainers saw). The unprepared trainer then lets the child know exactly what he or she is expected to do: reach a special state, called the "delta state." The trainer tells the child, while he is in the trance state, that he will know when he will reach it by the readings of the electrodes.

The trainer will tell the alter child, who has been called upon to be a "model" or building block for the new system, that delta is a good thing. He will emphasize this point repeatedly. The child will then be shocked to increase his receptivity to learning. This also wakes the child from his drugged state and he will be more alert. He will want to please the trainer. The trainer will tell the child that he wants him to perform certain mental exercises. The trainer will then give the child countdown exercises, which are used to help the child reach deeper trance states. Other verbal cues may be given to get the child into a trance. When the preparator or technical trainer sees delta waveforms, he or she signals the verbal trainer with a hand movement. The verbal trainer will immediately reward the child by saying, "good, you are in delta now". The trainer pats the child and tells him/her that he/she is doing a good job. If the child goes out of delta, the verbal trainer immediately becomes stern and shocks the child as punishment. The child is told that he or she has left the delta state (which is "good") and must return.

The induction, the counting, will be repeated until the delta state is again observed, when the child is repeatedly rewarded for entering that state and then staying there for longer and longer periods of time. Trainers use biofeedback principles to teach the child to consistently orient to a brainwave pattern. When the pattern can consistently stay in the delta pattern, it is rewarded. This process takes place over several months.

The trainers then have a model that still remains in a delta state, which they can begin to divide and use as a basis for forming a new system within. To do this, they will use the tools of drugs, hypnosis and trauma. The new system created will record delta waves on an EEG if done correctly. The new system learns what Delta means. Trainers often flash a delta signal or symbol (triangle) on an overhead projector, and "mold" the delta imprint. They wear robes with delta signs and dress the subject in clothes or robes with the delta sign. They teach the alters, under hypnosis, what the deltas do, how they act. They reward them when they comply and shock or traumatize them if they don't act like "deltas." They will give them jobs as deltas. They will watch high frequency movies that show delta functions. They can build a computer structure to contain the system, showing images of its organization while the subject is in a deep trance, having wiped the slate clean through trauma.

Here are some examples of how delta programming can be induced.

Other brainwave states will be induced in a similar way. They will often be formed from models that are extremely young internal children, which may be basic splits of splits, as the basis for programming. Commonly used brainwave states are

Alpha: This is the easiest brainwave state to reach, and it also includes the youngest and most easily accessible alters in the entire system. Young children have long periods of alpha activity and must be trained to enter other brainwave states for long periods of time. System access programming: access codes and sex alters are often placed in alpha, which may also be red coded in some systems.

Beta: This is the next easiest state to reach, and is often associated with aggressive impulses. The Beta state often contains cult protectors, internal warriors, and military systems. They can be coded blue.

Gamma: These are often extremely cult-like alters, and are more emotional than the other states, with the exception of alpha. The suicide program is often built into this system, as these alters would rather die than leave their "family". This system may contain erudition programs, as they memorize easily by heart. Multiple languages can be spoken by different alters in this system, as the Illuminati like to program in plural linguality, with up to eight languages, both modern and ancient, spoken.

Delta: This is one of the most cognitive brainwave states, often very dissociated. It can also be the "dominant" or controlling state of the other brainwave systems. Often the delta state can be configured internally as a computer, and delta alters will have flat, emotionless alters with photographic memories. They may hold most of the cognitive memories of other systems, especially if extensive amnesic programming has been done. The delta state can have up to three levels of training: delta 1, delta 2, and delta 3, which also corresponds to the security access allowed within the cult, i.e., access to highly confidential information. This system may contain behavioral science programs. Internal programmers, self-destruct, psychotic and destructive programs, and other sequences of punishment programs to prevent external or internal access to the systems may be held by the delta systems. It can be color coded orange/blue/purple and will often be the pathway to higher systems such as jewelry or internal councils.

Epsilon: This is often a "hidden system" that may contain CIA and high-level government programs. The assassin program may be in this system or in the beta system, depending on the trainer. Covert operations, courier operations, learning how to tail a subject, disguises, getting out of difficult situations can be handled by this system, which considers itself a chameleon. It can have a brown color code.

Phi/Theta/Omega programming: This is negative spiritual programming. These are the "dark" ritual alters, who participate in blood rituals, sacrifices and ceremonies. Internal witches, wizards, psychics, mediums, readers and practitioners of the occult will be placed in this system, which has a highly developed right brain and deep trance abilities. They are often coded in black.

This is an overview of the most common brainwave systems. It is often implemented over a period of years, from 8 to 21 years for the first ones, with occasional reinforcement of the programming from time to time.

Suggestions

Brainwave programming is a very complex form of programming that creates automatic amnesia and communication barriers between different brainwave states. This programming will also be reinforced by shocks and punishments to prevent its "degradation" or cancellation. The controllers and programmers of the internal system will also work to reinforce the programming, especially at night when the person is (physically) asleep.

All brainwave systems will have system controllers, usually organized in groups of three (the Illuminati like triads, as they are the "mystical" and most stable number. With the help of a good therapist, the survivor must learn about the controllers and communicators of the internal system. They are there, they have to be there, because the trainers put them there to communicate with and report to them externally, and they often have complete knowledge of their own system. They will also be fairly flat and disassociated from the knowledge of their own pain or the abuse that created them. This is a distancing mechanism, and the person's survival depended on their controller's ability to do this at any given time. She will often be very hostile and unwilling to look at her own abuse; she will become indignant at the thought and claim that she is cognitive and "above" the abuse (another lie told to her by her abusers).

Time, patience, discovering their needs, listening to them express their frustration, showing them the reality (i.e., that the controllers and all parties are related to each other, are part of the same person, and were ALL abused even though they may have disassociated from their pain), and trying to help them meet their needs for recognition, acceptance, and approval will begin to allow them to question their previous loyalty. These systems are often driven by fear: fear of punishment, fear of remembering (they were often the most tortured systems of the survivor and were promised amnesia in exchange for continued cooperation). Their fears are real and should be listened to and respected, as bursting and flooding programs are real threats to the survivor and can result in loss of functionality.

Flood programming is a sequence set up to punish a system if its internal programming is allowed to degrade or if access to an unauthorized person is allowed, either internally or externally. It involves fragments that hold very traumatic memories, both emotional and physical, being pushed forward and the person being "flooded" with wave after wave of memories. If this happens, and it often does if the survivor is in therapy, the first priority should be to slow down the memories. This may mean trying to reason with the internal controllers or deltas that allow the flooding; they need to know that if the front, or previously amnesiac alters, collapse, or are broken again due to the trauma, all systems will be weakened.

Negotiate with them. Prayer is helpful in this situation. Physical safety, including inpatient therapy, may be necessary if the flooding or bursting programs are activated. External physical safety is paramount for the survivor, who must be externally accountable as he or she defends against these intense program sequences. Frequent orientation to reality, explanation of new and more interesting jobs can be helpful. Undoing brainwave programming should ideally only be done with significant and safe external support, which may include additional therapy sessions, hospitalization if programming that could lead to loss of functionality or suicide is triggered, and should focus on improving internal communication and cooperation. The tasks of the alters can be changed: internal programmers can become internal deprogrammers; internal destroyers or punishers can become internal protectors; internal reporters who report to the cult can be asked to report internally on what the body is doing, and to keep it safe.

Here are some examples of possible changes. Befriend the system controllers, as they can become valuable helpers and will work with the therapist to keep the survivor safe.

CHAPTER SEVEN

Military programming

I would like to devote an entire chapter to military programming and the way it is carried out. Why? As we saw in Chapter 3, the Illuminati are increasingly emphasizing the importance of military training as part of their plan to take over. All of the children of the current generation are undergoing some form of military training as part of this plan.

Military training starts very early. It often begins at the age of three with simple drills. Children are taken by their parents to a training area, which may be a large auditorium indoors, or a remote area outdoors where training maneuvers are conducted. Tents are set up with command centers for the various military commanders and trainers.

Children are taught to walk in a rhythm, keeping a straight line. They are punished by being kicked, hit with a cattle prod or beaten with a club if they stray from their position. They will be dressed in small uniforms to mimic the adults.

Adults are given ranks, badges, and insignia indicating their level of achievement in the cult and military hierarchy. Badges and medals are given out to indicate the person's level of training and the tests they have passed. Commanders are often brutal and teach even the youngest children with harsh measures.

Children will be required to walk long distances, which increase as they grow, in all weather conditions. They must learn to overcome obstacles. They will be given "dummy" weapons, blank, when they are young. These weapons are perfect replicas of real weapons, but they fire blanks. Children learn to load and fire all kinds of guns, real and pretend, under close adult supervision. They will spend hours learning to aim and shoot at targets. At first, the targets are bull's-eyes, but as the children get older, the targets look like human silhouettes cut out by the police. Children learn to aim for the head or heart. Later, they will switch to realistic dummies. They are thus conditioned to kill a human being.

They will be shown violent war films, much more explicit and graphic than the usual group class films. Killing techniques will be shown in slow motion. The "kill or be killed" motif will be repeated over and over again. The trainer will ask the children what mistakes were made by those killed. Being killed is considered a weakness; being a killer is considered a strength.

At the age of seven or eight, children will be forced to crawl on their stomachs with simulated blanks fired over their heads. They are not told that these are blanks and they are extremely painful if the child is hit in the back or buttocks. They quickly learn to duck under fire. Combat conditions will be simulated as the children go through the years of "boot camp" training.

They will be rewarded with merit badges for good results, such as completing an obstacle course or maintaining composure under enemy fire. In other words, the cult creates a microcosm of real military training for its children and youth. Nazi concentration camps will be simulated, complete with guards and prisoners. The "guards" are usually older children or well-behaved youth. The "prisoners" are younger children or those who are punished for performing the maneuvers badly. There is a lot of pressure to want to be a guard and not be a prisoner, as prisoners are locked up, beaten, kicked, and made fun of.

Hunting and tracking games, for which prisoners are given half an hour of freedom, are common. These games may also involve the use of specially trained dogs to stun the prey, but not to kill it. Older children learn how to handle and use the dogs. Youngsters learn to help adults train the dogs.

Teenagers may be rewarded by becoming "youth leaders" who are allowed to plan the week's activities. Military training will closely follow the principles of Nazi military training and SS training. The trainers often spoke in German to the children, who had to learn the language. All commanders and senior adults speak German during these exercises. They may also speak French, as language skills are encouraged in the Illuminati.

Exercises for older youth include games where groups compete and the older teen leads, with the help of an adult advisor. Winning groups are rewarded; losing groups are punished. Youth learn to drop weak or slow members. Unfit members are shot or killed, and the youth leader is taught how to perform these tasks. They are taught to lead their unit in simulated battles with other units, and cold, cognitive logic under these conditions is rewarded. The goal is to create cognitive leaders within military systems who are dissociated from emotions under the stress of combat conditions.

The youth and their supporters are trained in all methods of crowd control. They watch special films that deal with all the possible reactions to a military takeover and the response of the crowd. These situations are then acted out in exercises, and the older youth leaders and their units are expected to deal with the various reactions. The "crowd" is trained by their trainers to act in different ways.

The ultimate goal of all this is to create an organized army of children, youth and adults who will know exactly what to do in the next world takeover. The training I have described is taking place not only in the United States, but in every country in the world. The best training centers are in Germany, Belgium, France and Russia. Military trainers are often sent to these countries to learn new techniques before being sent back to their home countries.

What to do:

It is important to understand that the military alters inside are extremely hierarchical. They are often internally ranked, with lower "foot soldiers" reporting to internal alters of increasing rank. In general, the higher the military rank, the higher the alter is in the system. A soldier without rank may not have much knowledge or influence on the system. His or her only job is to blindly obey others, after years of conditioning.

Inside officers often draw inspiration from outside authors, officers, or trainers. An officer

Generals often have much more knowledge than lower-ranking soldiers, and should be befriended because they can help with therapy.

It will take time, effort, and patience for the survivor and therapist to get to know these military officers. They are often abrupt, arrogant and extremely hostile to therapy. They are often very loyal to the cult and proud of their badges, awards, and accomplishments that have been earned after years of trauma and hard work. They are often reluctant to give these up because of the "loss" they perceive in leaving the cult.

They will also be surrounded by strong programming, including suicidal "honor/dishonor" programming (the brave and honorable soldier will die rather than betray his group, etc.) It is important to address the suicidal programming and intense limbic conditioning that many of these alters have been subjected to, while reasoning with the higher ranking members.

They will have a photographic memory and remember all aspects of military history. Providing them with safe and appropriate physical activities during the day can help them blow off steam. They are very physically prepared alters, who enjoy running, walking, and target practice with guns and knives. It may be helpful to let them go hiking (with a trusted person) and allow them to practice outdoor activities.

Acknowledging their importance to the survivor and the trauma they have experienced, respecting their loyalty, bravery, and appealing to their sense of honor to help the system stay safe (these alters often have a highly developed, if misguided, sense of honor) can be helpful. Internal praise for bravery, or even an internal award ceremony (they are used to this) for parties who have decided to leave the cult and protect the body, can be arranged. They are used to praise and recognition for a job well done, and need that motivation. They were used to receiving this from the cult, but the survivor may turn the locus of control inward, rather than outward, in order to break ties with the cult.

Military protectors can change their job to keep the body safe from attackers. They can be the best asset in a system, as they are very good at "kicking ass" and are not easily scared off. They may be able to tell outside attackers to leave the survivor alone and protect the survivor from outside access.

It is also helpful to allow them to express their feelings through therapy, journaling, photos and collages. Although high-ranking officers are often very disassociated from their feelings, they can begin to empathize with those below them who have endured their pain and the weight of brutal and punitive experiences. They must be willing to acknowledge that they have been abused at some point, that they have been deceived and used. Seeking out the younger alters from whom they were separated will help them in this process. With time and good internal communication, as well as patience on the part of the therapist and the survivor, military alters can become one of the best assets and allies in staying safe from cults.

CHAPTER EIGHT

CIA, government and scholarship programs

Some systems have internal CIA programming. Some of the methods mentioned in previous chapters, such as brainwave programming and color coding, were developed in part with CIA funding in the 1950s and 1960s. Military intelligence officers working in Langley, Virginia, used these government funds to conduct research on human subjects. They shared what they were learning with trainers in the United States and Europe.

CIA programming can include alters in a system trained in various techniques to find a target and study it without being detected. The end result of marking the victim may be a sexual relationship with the target, or people within the system trained in the assassination of a target.

These are complex programming sequences, set up after years of training, with periodic reinforcements. Alters can be trained to become hyper-aware of their surroundings and able to hear whispered conversations. Internal recorders are trained to download these conversations, along with other information. The emphasis is on photographic recall, as the person is hypnotized or put into a delta state to "download" information to the trainer or CIA agent.

The CIA-programmed survivor will have received extensive training in how to "drop a beacon" (detect anyone following them and abandon them). This training begins in early childhood and continues as the child grows. Children are often taken to a neutral-colored training room. They may be drugged or hypnotized, usually a combination of both.

They will be shown training films on how a CIA agent works. They will be told that they are "special," "chosen," "one in a thousand" who is the only one who can do this special job. They are told that they are becoming a secret CIA agent. The young child, who has no idea what the CIA is, focuses on the fact that he has been chosen because he is special, that he is needed and that he will be eager to please. The child is taken to a dinner or play organized by the trainer. There will be a group of ten to sixteen people at the "party. Afterwards, the child will be questioned at length by the trainer. Who was sitting where? What clothes were they wearing? What color were their eyes? What color were their eyes? What color was their hair? Who gave the speech? What did they say? The child will be praised if he or she answers correctly, but punished and shocked if he or she is unable to remember the details. This is to reinforce the natural photographic memory and help the child record the details. The next few times, the child's abilities will improve as he or she wants to avoid punishment.

In the next level of training, the child will be asked to observe and understand: Who is the most important person in the room? Why? The child will be taught body movements and mannerisms that give non-verbal cues. The child can be taught to approach important adults or a designated target, first in a role-playing game and then in real life, and engage them in casual conversation while seeking out information that they have been instructed to obtain. They can be taught to be innocently attractive, and they will be dressed accordingly. They are often taught to lure the target into having sex with them.

An older youth, or adult, will learn not only to lure a target into bed, but also to kill them, if they are a target for assassination, while they are sleeping or relaxing after sex. They are taught to search the target's belongings for any information the trainer or cult leader needs. Often, before being tasked with an assassination, the cult member is indoctrinated on why killing the victim is a service to humanity. He will be lied to about being the head of a pornography ring, a pedophile or a brutal villain. This will arouse the killer's natural anger toward the person and motivate him, while helping him to overcome his natural moral reluctance and guilt about killing a human being.

They will learn to disguise themselves, changing clothes, gender (pretending to be the opposite sex), makeup, contact lenses, and how to get out of the situation safely. They will learn to overcome interrogation techniques through extensive training and hypnosis, in case they get caught. They will learn to self-suicide with a pill or a dagger, if they are arrested, in most cases.

Suggestions

CIA programming involves the use of sophisticated technology to enhance its effectiveness and can be difficult to break. It may involve the person being traumatized in isolation tanks (which will also be done with brainwave programming). It may involve sensory deprivation, sensory overload, isolation, sleep deprivation. It can be a matter of listening for hours to repetitive tapes in headphones. The subject is shocked or severely punished if they try to remove the headphones. They are hypnotized, tortured, subjected to various combinations of drugs, exposed to harmonic sounds, often in one ear or the other. They will be exposed to flashing strobe lights, which can cause seizures, and the alters will be programmed to cause seizures if the subject tries to break the programming. They will be shown high-speed movies with different tracks, one for the left eye and one for the right eye, to increase brain division or dichotomous thinking.

The survivor and the therapist must work slowly to undo the effects of this trauma. The person will have to accept, slowly and carefully, how the programming was done. They may have to learn their own access codes (the same goes for brainwaves and other sophisticated programming techniques). They will have to communicate with the alters and traumatized fragments inside, let them know that they have been used. They will have to help the young alters, who were divided to create the system, and who have often suffered the worst trauma. Grieving the abuse, trauma, methodical calculations and scientific methods used to set up this programming will take time. It will be important to let go of the feelings, including rage, in a safe way. The survivor may be afraid of strong feelings and will particularly fear anger and rage, as they will associate these feelings with the need to kill, hurt or murder others. It is important to let the feelings come out slowly and carefully, knowing that homicidal and suicidal feelings are likely to arise.

If the ability to control acting out is a problem, the client may need to be hospitalized in a secure facility that includes mind control and cult programs. He will fear being labeled "psychotic" because the programmers have told him he will be called that and locked up forever. The WORST thing a therapist or hospital can do in this situation is to play on these fears or label the person as psychotic. It is important to constantly ground the person in reality, using anchoring exercises, to slowly and carefully release feelings of rage and betrayal, to constantly reinforce the idea that the person can remember and not become psychotic or die, to believe in and value the person. The survivor may exhibit unstable behavior at times, but this is not psychosis, but rather a natural reaction to extreme trauma. The survivor needs to realize this and know that he or she can overcome the effects with time and good therapy. They will need hope and a good support system.

Government programming

Government programs involve training for leadership or administrative positions in government. He or she may be trained to network with other members of local, national and international governments. The stated goal of the Illuminati is to infiltrate all major governments in the world and ultimately bring about their downfall. Government agents learn to do this by infiltrating local political parties, running for local and national elections, working for key leaders, as administrators, financial advisors, funding government races and supporting the Illuminati-friendly person, or placing their person to win, creating political chaos and unrest through agents trained in dissent. Those selected for government programs are usually highly intelligent and have natural charm or charisma. They are also skilled manipulators. These abilities can be enhanced by programming, encouraging the person to project a "persona" that will attract people to them.

They are also taught finances extensively. This programming is done by hypnotizing the person, whether a child, youth, or adult (it is usually initiated in late childhood in suitable candidates), and inducing a deep trance with drugs. The person is shocked and then informed of the trainer's and the cult's agenda towards them. She is told that she is very special to the Illuminati and that she will be one of the people who will help change world history. She is told that she will be rewarded with wealth, popularity and power for carrying out the cult's agenda. They are told and shown the punishment for disobedience. They are shown training films on government, how it works, national and international affairs. They meet with special teachers who train them in the internal political workings of the group they want to infiltrate, including the power structure and the strengths and weaknesses of key players.

They will learn all the languages needed for the job. They will go to university or receive the training and education necessary to be credible. They will receive special scholarships to fund these studies, if necessary.

They have the opportunity to practice their skills in infiltration, information gathering, manipulation of people and politics in a staged setting and later in real life situations. If they need to learn how to control the media, they will learn the methods to do so. They receive extensive support and mentoring throughout their careers.

Suggestions

Government programming is quite complex, as it is related to the natural abilities of the individual. It can be difficult for people to detach themselves from the role they are playing and often only feel acceptable when they are doing their job. They may find it difficult to believe that their careers, friendships, marriages and contacts have been secretly guided by the cult for most of their lives. They may feel offended, betrayed or angry when they realize this. It will also be difficult for them not to use the manipulative techniques that come so naturally to them, both on their therapist and on themselves, to ease the pain that the truth may cause. The person and alters who have undergone this type of programming have a lot to lose if they abandon their role and persona, and must count the cost of leaving and recognize the difficulty of doing so. They will have to grieve for having been used and for the false interpretation of reality they have believed in all their lives. Listening to the other parts of the person and acknowledging the reality of cult abuse will be important steps in breaking free. Achieving a new career in the person's life will also help restore a shattered self-image.

Scholarship training

The Illuminati revere scholarship, especially the oral tradition. Children with good memory and native intelligence can be specifically trained in scholarship. This will include trauma-induced learning, with praise for success. It will also involve punishment or shock for poor performance. The main areas of scholarship include:

Oral tradition: history of the Illuminati, especially the particular branch of the child, memorization of genealogies. Learning and mastering several languages, modern and ancient, including but not limited to: English, French, German, Russian, Spanish, Arabic, Latin, Greek, Hebrew, Egyptian hieroglyphics, ancient Babylonian, ancient Chaldean and cuneiform writings. Some revered ancient texts are written in very ancient languages, and some ceremonies may include rituals that use them. Learn ancient and modern history and become skilled at planning role plays and dramatizations. Learn to teach others the skills mentioned above. The child who becomes a scholar is also expected to become a competent teacher and pass on his knowledge to others. He or she will practice teaching in the classroom and in one-on-one sessions.

Suggestions

Fellowship programs involve alters who are intensely loyal to the cult, as they believe they are connected to a long, unbroken lineage of people from the beginning of history. They are often immersed in the philosophy of the cult, having read and memorized many esoteric volumes related to it. Appealing to their logic, intellect, and open-mindedness and discussing with them the pros and cons of leaving the cult will often be well received. They despise open conflict and prefer to approach problems intellectually. They are good at debating and are very vocal. Asking them to read books that deal with liberation from the cult, and asking them to witness and listen to the stories of traumatized alters, whether in their system or inside, will often help them make the decision to change loyalties. Although they have been immersed in false ideologies and doctrines, they are often willing to be intellectually honest. They read and debate both sides of an issue and may be among the first to make the decision to leave the cult once they are convinced that it is abusive.

CHAPTER NINE

Programming related to stories, movies, cartoons or role-playing games

In this chapter, I want to discuss a particular type of programming that is universal among the Illuminati. This is programming that is tied to a story, movie, cartoon or role-playing game.

For countless centuries, Illuminati trainers and leaders have used role-playing to reinforce and program children, and it is still a favorite mode of instruction today. A typical role-play involves a "visit back in time." The child is told, while drugged or hypnotized, that he or she and the other children accompanying him or her (usually a small group goes through this program together) are going to travel back in time. The trainer or teacher is seen as immensely powerful by the children, as he or she magically transports them back in time. They enter another room, where people are dressed in period costumes from the historical period the teacher wants the children to learn about. Everything is historically accurate and well documented. For example, if the children are to visit ancient Rome, they will be taken to a Senate room, where the characters are dressed in togas. They speak to each other in ancient Latin and debate issues. Caesar, or another king will enter the Senate. Roman customs for a scenario like this will be followed throughout the roleplay.

One of the goals of this role-playing game is to give children a look behind the scenes of history. The Illuminati agenda will be highlighted and children will "see" that famous people in history were actually Illuminists. This will reinforce their "specialness" and the historicity of the group. It will also reinforce language learning, as the scenes may take place in medieval England, or the French court of Louis XIV, etc. The scenes will also contain a moral that will build on the programming the children have been following. Perhaps they will see a "traitor" being "guillotined" at the French court. Or an unworthy senator, who tries to betray his king, will be stabbed. The child may be given a role in the play, such as carrying a secret message to the king or queen, to reinforce the courier schedule. The child truly believes that he or she has entered the story and is part of the process of creating the story.

In modern times, programming has become more sophisticated with the advent of technology. Before television or movies, programs were often "scripted" around famous fairy tales or stories, read aloud by one trainer while the second trainer worked with the child. A "reader" must have a good singing voice. The child is read the story and, under hypnosis and trauma, is told that he is one of the characters in the story. The "real" meaning of the story, its "hidden meaning," is explained to him and he is told that every time he hears the story, he must remember what it really means.

Today, movies and videos are frequently used in programming. Favorite scripts include: Walt Disney movies (Disney was an Illuminati), especially Fantasia, Sleeping Beauty, The Little Mermaid, Cinderella, Beauty and the Beast. The Wizard of Oz, both the books and the movie were used. Any film incorporating illuminist themes can be used. E.T. and Star Wars have been used in recent years.

How is the programming of the scripts done?

The trainer plays the film for the child. The child is informed that he or she will be "asked about" the film, which encourages the child to use photographic recall of what he or she sees. The trainer can show the child a shortened version of the film, with only parts of the whole, or can show the child a short scene from the film.

After watching the movie or scene, the child is drugged to relax, and then asked what he or she remembers. The child will be shocked if he or she does not remember what the trainer feels is important, and will be forced to watch the scenes repeatedly.

When the child remembers the segments perfectly, the trainer tells the child that this is one of the characters. The child may be highly traumatized at first, and a blank personality is created inside to become the desired character. The first thing the blank slate sees is a recording of the movie or scene. This is its "first memory". The trainer then associates the scene with Illuminati ideology. The trainer will teach the child the "hidden meaning" of the film and congratulate him or her for being one of the few "enlightened ones" to understand what it really means. Script programming is often linked to other programming that the child is experiencing. Military programming may be linked to Star Wars. Total recall programming can be linked to Data in Star Trek.

Computer programming can be linked to Hal in 2001 A Space Odyssey; internal maze programming can be linked to the movie "Labyrinth." The possibilities are wide-ranging and depend on both the child and the trainer as to where the programming of the scenario will go. The music of the program or scene will be used as a trigger to access the inner programming or to bring out these personalities.

Suggestions

Scripted programming often involves a great deal of trauma in order to create the desired "blank slate" alterations. The programming will be anchored by repetition, electroshock, torture, drugs and hypnosis. Alters who have undergone this programming are often very disconnected from external reality and may believe that they are part of a "script." They may be Dorothy in search of the Emerald City (or the completion of Illuminati domination of the earth). They can be a computer or the character Data. Reality orientation will be very important. Allow these parts to experience a safe external reality and check for themselves if they are really part of a man or woman. Looking in the mirror can be helpful when they express a desire to do so. The presence of cognitive assistants who can share with them memories of everyday life can help them to anchor themselves in reality. At first, they will be very surprised, even indignant or hostile, when it is suggested that they are not the character. They will think that the therapist is a trainer or part of the scenario, since this is the only reality they have known. It will be necessary to patiently bring them back, again and again, to the present reality, to increase communication with others within, and finally to grieve the intense amount of deception and deception they have experienced. With time and patience, these parts will be willing to let go of their old "scripted" roles and become part of the person's present reality.

CHAPTER TEN

The sixth stage of the discipline: betrayal; twinning, internal walls, structures, geometry

This chapter addresses the sixth stage of discipline in the Illuminati:

Programming of betrayal

The programming of betrayal will begin in infancy, but will become formalized around the age of six or seven and will continue into adulthood. The sixth stage can be summarized as follows: "betrayal is the greatest good". Illuminati teach this to their children as a very important spiritual principle. They idealize treachery as the true state of man. The keen mind, the follower, quickly learns this and learns to manipulate it.

The child will learn this principle through a series of set-ups. The child will be placed in situations where an adult who is kind and who, in a series of enactments, "saves" the child gains the child's trust. The child sees the adult as a "savior" after the adult has intervened and protected him/her repeatedly. After months or even a year of bonding, the child turns to the adult for help one day. The adult backs down, mocks the child, and begins to abuse the child. This sets up the following programming: adults will always betray a child and other adults.

Another pattern will involve twinning, which deserves special mention here. The Illuminati often create twin bonds in their children. The ideal is to have identical twins, but this is not always possible. So the child is allowed to play with and bond with another child in the cult from an early age. At some point, the child learns that the other child is actually his or her "twin" and was separated at birth. He or she is told that this is a big secret and that he or she must not tell anyone or he will be punished. The child, who is often alone and isolated, is overjoyed. He has a twin, someone who has a special bond with him because of his birth.

The children do everything together. They go to school together, do military training together. They tell each other secrets. They are also often friends during the day. They are taught to cross paths with each other, like real siblings would.

But at some point, they will be forced to hurt each other. If one of the "twins" is considered expendable, the ultimate scenario will be when one twin is forced to die in front of the other. One twin may collect secrets from the other twin, be forced to reveal them to a coach or cult leader, and then be forced to kill the other twin. One twin can be forced to hit or hurt the other. If he or she refuses, the other twin will be brutalized by the trainer and the twin who refused will be told that the child was injured because of his or her refusal to comply. In many cases, one twin is forced to betray the other and turn against him or her after intensive programming. This betrayal will devastate both children, and they will learn the real lesson: trust no one. Betray or be betrayed.

Children will also have adult role models in every hand, as the cult is a very political, hierarchical, backstabbing society. Adults are constantly betraying each other, stepping over each other to move up. Children will see an adult being praised, advanced, because he or she betrayed others below them, or set them up to fail. Children quickly learn to imitate the adults around them, and both adults and children can become quite cynical about human nature. They will have seen it at its worst, whether it be in training sessions, the brutality of a commander in the military, or the gossip and backstabbing that occurs before and after rituals. They also integrate the message internally: play the game or get crushed. Even the youngest children learn to manipulate others at an early age, while adults laugh at how quickly they learn the ways of adults. Manipulating people is considered an art in the cult, and those who practice it best, as in any group, often win.

Suggestions

The betrayal program may have completely broken the survivor's trust in outsiders. It will take a long, long time for the therapist to gain the survivor's trust. These are people who have been taught over and over that talking, sharing secrets would be severely punished. The little ones inside will be very cautious at first, not believing that the therapist is not just another trainer who will one day yell "aha!" and betray them if they start to trust. This trust takes time and patience, and must be earned through sessions where the therapist shows that they are trustworthy and not abusive. Survivors will test therapists over and over again to see if they are really who they say they are. This is a normal part of the therapeutic process. Survivors may even try to turn away from therapy or outside support, as genuine caring support will cause them to "come out of the woodwork," meaning it will conflict incredibly with their worldview and experiences before leaving the cult.

The survivor and therapist need to understand that some distrust is healthy, based on what the survivor has experienced, and can be life-saving, helping to protect the survivor from outside access. Honor this need and be patient while the survivor tests again and again. The survivor may try to reason with the inner alters who have been betrayed to the point of legitimate paranoia. They can ask them to observe and see what the therapist and/or support person looks like. To take their time, to examine them. To be aware that what they have experienced may amplify normal feelings of caution. By helping them to orient themselves to the external reality, and in particular to positive experiences where they have some confidence and are not hurt, it will be possible to make great progress in resolving this problem. The survivor may feel confusion and internal conflict when experiencing a world where trust is possible. He or she may pull away or, conversely, become very dependent on the therapist and share his or her experience too quickly because of a desire for safe intimacy that was never satisfied. Setting healthy boundaries while acknowledging needs will help the survivor through this stage.

Another type of programming involves the deliberate creation of internal structures within the cult member.

Internal structures: temples, eyes, mirrors, carousels, etc.

Illuminati trainers will try to create internal structures in the person's personality systems. Why? They believe it creates more stability. It also gives the alters and fragments a place to hang out inside, and creates a convenient way to call them. If a fragment is indexed inside an internal helix, for example, the trainer knows how to locate them more easily.

Internal structures vary considerably depending on the trainer, the group, the region of the United States or Europe, and the goals of the individual. Common internal structures include, but are not limited to, the following

> **Temples:** these are often dedicated to the main Illuminati deities and spiritual altars gather there. They may be real temples, Masonic or private, which the subject may have visited.

> **The temple of Moloch** will be created in black stone with a fire burning inside.

> **All-seeing Eye of Horus:** one of the most common structures in an Illuminati system; universal. Horus is a deity worshipped by the Illuminati, and the all-seeing eye internally represents the fact that the sect can always see what the individual is doing. It also represents having been given to Horus in a great ceremony. The eye can be closed or open, depending on the state of the system at the time. This eye will also be linked to demonic surveillance of the person's activities at any given time.

> **Pyramids:** The Illuminati revere ancient Egyptian symbology, especially the "mystery religion" and the teachings of the Temple of Set. Pyramids will be placed inside, both for stability (a triangle and/or pyramid represent strength and stability) and as a place to call the demons. Pyramids and triangles, along with the number three, represent the call to the demon in Illuminist philosophy.

> **Sun:** represents Ra, the sun god

> **Geometric figures:** configurations of circles, triangles, pentagons, etc. Geometric patterns are considered sacred and are based on an ancient philosophy. There may be hundreds of them overlapping in a training grid for complex systems, which will house fragments in each of them.

> **Training grids:** these can be simplistic, such as patterned cubes, rows of boxes, or more complex, such as helixes, double helixes, infinite loops. Each trainer will have favorites categorized as

simple, medium, and complex, depending on the child and their ability to remember and memorize.

➢ **Columns:** Greek Doric columns, Ionic columns. They are often used in "time travel" programs, with a portal between two columns.

➢ **Computers:** complex systems, highly dissociated, with alters and fragments kept in a computer system.

➢ **Robots:** they can be present in older systems

➢ **Crystals:** gems, balls, multi-faceted. Used in spiritual systems to enhance occult powers. Alters and fragments can gather on the facets of a large ball.

➢ **Mirrors:** used internally to reinforce other programming sequences, internal twinning and distortion of reality programming. Can create shadow systems of functional systems. Can also lock in demonic programming.

➢ **Carousels:** used in some programming sequences to confuse the alters inside. Often related to spinning, programming confusion inside. Can be used to punish internal alters; they will be turned on the carousel if they say so.

➢ **Playing cards:** these can be cards from a deck of cards or complex configurations consisting of hundreds of cards inside. The programming of dominoes is similar. All dominoes touch each other and if someone tries to dismantle the programming, the deck will fall.

➢ **Black Boxes:** represent self-destruct and bursting programs sealed in a black box to protect the system. It should not be opened without careful preparation and good therapy.

➢ **Mines, traps:** see above

➢ **Spider webs:** represent linked programming, with a spider (internal programmer) continually weaving the web and reinforcing internal programming and punishments. The web also communicates with other systems. It can also represent internal demonic links, woven within.

➢ **Internal training rooms:** used as punishment for internal alters. Will represent the external training rooms that the person went to.

➤ **Internal walls:** they often represent very large internal amnesia barriers. Walls can be very thick, impermeable or semi-permeable. A typical use of a wall will be to maintain high levels of amnesia between the amnesic alters of the "front" or daily life, and the active alters of the "back" or cult, which contains more information about the person's life history. The back may be able to selectively see over the wall and go through it, but the front will be completely unaware that there is a wall or what is behind it.

➤ **Seals:** usually in groups of six or seven, they represent the demonic seal and can cover the end times, the collapse of programs, as well as the role within the sect in the new hierarchy.

These are some common programming structures. Again, there are many, many other types of internal structures, the number and type of which are limited only by the creative abilities of the trainer and the survivor.

The way these structures are placed in the person is quite similar. Under the effect of drugs, hypnosis or electroshock, the person is traumatized and placed in a deep trance state. In this state of deep trance, he or she is asked to open his or her eyes and look at: either a projected image of the structure, or a 3D model of it, or a holographic image using a virtual reality helmet. The image will be brought closer, using shocks and bringing the image closer to the person's visual field. It can be rotated, if graphics are available, or a 3D image is used. The person can be told that they are going inside, if it is a temple or pyramid, under deep hypnosis, that they (the programmed alter) will now "live inside" the structure, box, map, etc. This will also serve to reinforce the programming of amnesia and isolation within, as the structure will be used to reinforce the walls between the alter/fragment and other alters and fragments within.

Suggestions

If the survivor finds structures inside, it will first be helpful to try to understand WHY they are there. What is their purpose? To reinforce amnesia? Isolation? Spiritual programming? Punishment? To contain dangerous programming sequences? This question is important because some structures such as internal walls or barriers may have been created not only by the cult, but also reinforced by the survivor as a means of internal protection. The survivor may not want to dismantle the internal structures too quickly without knowing their purpose and what they contain. The survivor and therapist will need to go slowly. The first step will be to learn how the structures were put in place and what alters are connected to them. A long, slow, careful preparation, with a great deal of cooperation from the system, will be needed to examine some structures. This may only happen after years of intensive therapy. Each survivor will progress at his or her own pace. If a wall is present, breaking it down slowly, one brick at a time, or allowing part of it to become semi-permeable may be a first step toward healing. Equipment in training rooms can be turned off and taken down; the room can be turned into a safe room, redecorated and rearranged with toys and safe objects. Computers can slowly begin to realize that they are human and gradually be allowed to take on human characteristics.

Survivors can use their creativity to reclaim their person, with the support of their therapists, and undo what has been done.

CHAPTER ELEVEN

Suicidal programming

I have decided to write an entire chapter on suicidal programming, as this is often the most dangerous programming the survivor will face during their healing process. ALL ILLUMINATI SURVIVORS WILL HAVE SUICIDAL PROGRAMMING PROTECTING THEIR SYSTEM. I have emphasized this point to reiterate the need for good therapy and a strong support system for the survivor.

The Illuminati know and realize that over time, members of their group may begin to question what they are doing. They may also become disenchanted with their role. They may even want to leave the group or try to dismantle their own programming.

Trainers are well aware of this possibility and, to avoid it, they always program suicidality. Suicidality, or suicidal programming, can surround one or more systems internally. It can be superimposed on more than one system.

From early childhood, survivors have been conditioned to believe that they would rather die than leave their "family" (the Illuminati group). This is the core or foundation of suicidal programming. It will be closely tied to loyalty to the family and the group (remember, this is a generational group and leaving may mean giving up all contact with parents, spouses, siblings, aunts, uncles, cousins and children, as well as close friends). These people will all try to contact the survivor and lure him or her back into the cult, asking, "Don't you like us anymore?" and even becoming accusatory and hostile if the survivor does not respond as they wish. The survivor will be told that he or she is "crazy. Or that he is delusional. That his family loves him and would never be in a cult. The family members will all remain amnesiac, unless something triggers their own memories.

One of the most common suicidal programming sequences placed inside is the "come back or die" programming. A family member can activate it by telling the survivor that they miss him or her and that the family wants to see them. If the survivor does not return, the programming is turned on. It can only be deactivated by a code word from the person's trainer or cult contact person. This ensures that he or she will make contact again. If the survivor tries to break this programming, he or she will need help, both internal and external, for safety.

Hospitalization may be necessary in a secure facility that understands DID and programming, as well as suicidality, because the alters inside will begin to fight if the person tries to break the programming. They have been programmed to commit suicide, to be broken internally, or at the very least, to be severely punished, and they are afraid of the repercussions of not obeying. The survivor will need to get to know these internal alters and reassure them that they no longer need to do their job.

Suicidal timed programming is another type of internally placed program. It does not require contact with family members to be activated. In fact, it activates automatically after a period of time WITHOUT contact with the cult. Controlling alters and/or punishing alters will have been programmed to commit suicide if a certain period of time passes without contact with the trainer. They will be told that the only way to avoid this is to reconnect with the trainer, who knows a command code to stop the program. The time interval can range from three to nine months, as each system is different. Recall programs may have this as a backup to ensure compliance.

Layered systems programming is a particularly complex form of suicide programming in which multiple systems (up to six at a time) are programmed to simultaneously trigger suicide programming. This type of programming always requires hospitalization for the safety of the survivor.

Honor and dishonor programming is common in military systems. In this case, the military is told that an "honorable and courageous" soldier will commit suicide rather than reveal secrets or leave his unit.

The "Say Nothing" program is often reinforced by a suicidal program.

The denial of access program, which prevents unauthorized access to the exterior and interior, will often be reinforced by a suicide/homicide program or both.

Almost all suicide programs are set up to ensure continued obedience to the cult's program, to ensure regular reconnection, or to prevent the individual or an outsider from accessing the person's system without authorization (i.e., the correct access codes, which trainers are careful to use at the beginning of each session). It often blocks therapy, as the survivor is understandably terrified of dying if they reveal their inner world or story.

Suggestions

First, the survivor and therapist need to determine what suicidal programming is present (it is likely present, it is not necessary to ask IF it is present). Internal communication and discovery of the alters or fragments that contain the suicidal programming will be important. Physical safety, whether with a safe outsider or inpatient, while working on the suicide programming is extremely important, as the programming may lead the survivor to self-destructive behavior or back into the cult. Treatment of suicide programming requires that the survivor and therapist have a good internal communication system in place. This is extremely important, as the survivor will need internal cooperation to dismantle the suicidality.

Letting the inner alters know that they no longer have to do their job, that they can change, can be helpful. Reality orientation, letting them know that if they kill the body, they will die, can also help (often these parts have been fooled into believing that they will not die, if they do their job. So they need to hear the truth). Having control alters, high-level alters who have influence over the system, agree to help the therapist dismantle the programming can be helpful. But be aware that some internal suicide sequences will be set up that even the controllers cannot dismantle. Creating an internal safety committee whose main task is to ensure the safety of the body and to ask for help if the suicidal programming begins to set in, BEFORE THE ACT HAPPENS, will also be of great help.

As the survivor develops trust with their therapist and realizes the value of life, and that life can be much better than it ever was, they will become more willing to reach out and ask for help if they become suicidal. The survivor may also find that he or she is facing deep despair. This despair may have been used by the cult to set up a suicidal program, but it is not a program per se. A very young divided core may have taken on many of the feelings of hopelessness, helplessness, failure, and a desire to die that the child felt growing up in a horribly abusive atmosphere. These are not programming, but real feelings, and it will be important to differentiate them from the programming. If the basic despair appears, the alter that contains it may also state that it has been trained not to commit suicide or to give up. Trainers will do this if the despair begins to overwhelm the subject at an early age, in order to prevent the child's suicide.

The survivor's cognitives, helpers, and nurturers will all need to be brought together to help that part of the core heal. There will be intense, and legitimate, grief and anguish for the immense pain that the young child has endured. Despair will be expressed. It may be helpful for alters with happier memories to try to share their memories with this very young part. Outside support and attention can also make a big difference. Healing from the immense pain caused by this central split will take a long time and should not be rushed. Antidepressants can help, as depression can be shared by all systems. Messages of hope, new and positive experiences can help the survivor overcome this type of program, as can journaling, poetry, artwork and collage of feelings. Time, patience, support, the ability to express feelings safely, and physical safety if necessary will go a long way in helping the survivor overcome these issues.

CHAPTER TWELVE

Preventing access to the survivor

This chapter is by far one of the most important I have written in this book. Why? Deprogramming cannot be successful if the person is still in contact with their abusers.

Survivors take a step forward, only to find themselves internally defeated. All efforts in therapy will be undone or questioned. Survivors and their therapist will find that they are struggling to find internal alters. Entire systems may shut down. A child's presentation system may emerge.

Confusers and jammers will take control of the therapy sessions and blockers will block the therapy.

No chapter can ever be completely comprehensive on how to prevent re-contact. What I will share are some of the most common ways that the cult and trainers attempt to reaccess individuals, and I will give some techniques to prevent this.

The cult has a vested interest in keeping its members. After all, they have spent generations telling their members that if they left, they would die, be killed or become psychotic. It makes them very unhappy to see someone who is very much alive and clearly not psychotic leave. The most resistant members also question the veracity of what they have been told if they see someone leave. The departure of one member can break the hold some programs have on other members. Trainers especially hate to see someone leave and gnash their teeth on this issue at night. A member's departure from the cult is considered a failure of the training and trainers can be severely punished.

The cult has therefore found certain ways to keep its members with it, willingly or by force. These means include, but are not limited to:

E.T. phone home: the individual will have personalities whose only task is to call and report to the trainer or cult leader. These are often young children who just want to be satisfied, need attention and care and are highly rewarded when they call the cult leader back. Any survivor who tries to leave the cult is faced with the urge to call home. To call their abusers. To call their friends who are part of the group. To call their parents, siblings, cousins or aunts. This urge can sometimes become overwhelming, and worse, the survivor may be completely unaware that the people they are calling are cult members who are urging them, in code, to return. The most common phrases are: your "family" loves you, misses you, needs you. So-and-so is sick and needs to see you. You are so special to us. You are very valuable. You need to come see us. Why are you so distant? Why haven't we heard from you lately?

The list is long. Soft, gentle phrases with double meanings, placed in the person during training sessions. Trainers are not stupid and know that if cult members said "come to the ritual meeting at midnight next week," the survivor would run the other way and be confirmed that he or she is not making it up. So they insert coded messages behind innocuous phrases such as those described above.

These and other messages are intended to trigger recontact programming.

In recontact programming (ALL ILLUMINATI MEMBERS HAVE RECONTACT PROGRAMMING, IT IS NEVER LEFT TO CHANCE), the person has parts whose only job is to have contact with his or her trainer or the cult leader, or the person in charge (the person one rung above them in the cult). These parts are heavily programmed, through drugs, hypnosis, shocks, torture, to make contact again. The individual will feel agitated, shaky, weepy, scared if they try to break this programming. This programming is often linked or associated with suicidal programming (see previous chapter for more information on suicidal programming). She may exhibit symptoms of post-traumatic stress, even flooding programs and sequences of internal self-punishment, as she struggles internally with this programming.

Siblings are often cross-trained to access each other using special codes. Don't forget that... Can be the origin of this. The phrases "I love you" or "Your family loves you" can also be used. Phrases are personalized, based on family members and the person's background.

Certain clothing or jewelry worn can be used to emphasize a system of cult loyalty, such as a color-coded or jewelry system. The person must physically resemble the person assigned to them in the programming sequence, so that a person wearing a ruby pin, for example, will not inadvertently bring out alters. This type of cue will be based on visual recognition of a person, as well as the color of clothing or jewelry worn in a certain way.

Phone calls from concerned family members, friends, and cult members will flood the survivor's phone lines and answering machine, especially during the initial exit phase.

Hang-up calls, three or six in a row, or calls where a series of tones are heard can be used as cues to call the person back and trigger internal programming.

Birthday, vacation or "we miss you" cards or letters can be sent with trigger codes.

Flowers with a certain number of flowers or a certain color can be sent. Daisies can trigger internal programming.

The possibilities are almost endless, depending on the trainers, the group the person belonged to, and the people they are most connected to in the cult. Special training sessions will be held, with code words and clues built into the programming of the system.

If all else fails, hostility sets in. One will hear, "You don't like us," even though the survivor has repeatedly stated that he or she cares. Boundaries set with cult members will be interpreted as a lack of interest or withdrawal. Accusations, guilt and anger, and manipulation will be used as hooks to make the survivor feel guilty for withdrawing from the cult.

The isolation program may become active as the cult support system is removed from the survivor's life and the survivor strives to develop healthy and appropriate relationships outside the cult. Often, the therapist will be the survivor's lifeline and only support at first. The person may quickly fall into codependent relationships or relationships with other survivors to fill the void in their lives. In the worst case, desperate for care and feeling isolated, he or she will befriend the first caring person they meet. This person may be a cult member, sent to make a quick friendship. Survivors should be wary of "instant friendships" or instant connections with others. Most good relationships take time and effort.

Suggestions

One of the most difficult, but most important safety tasks will be for a total amnesiac presentation system to realize the identity of its abusers. It will seem unbelievable when back parts come forward in therapy and reveal that beloved, or even barely tolerated, family members are part of the cult. Believing these parts and listening to them will be crucial for safety. Protectors will be important to the survivor's safety, especially if they are willing to renounce their allegiance to the cult and help the person stay safe. External accountability to safe people is extremely important. The problem is that generational Illuminati survivors have often been surrounded their entire lives by a network of other cult members. Unbeknownst to them, their closest friends and family members are part of the group. Amnesia is the greatest danger to the survivor in the early stages, as they will trust people before they remember that they are not safe.

A survivor may remember that his father took him to rituals and believe that his mother or grandmother is safe. Only later, in therapy, will he or she remember that his or her mother or grandmother was actually his or her coach, as the most painful memories tend to come later. The survivor may only remember ritual abuse in early childhood and think that he or she was released at a certain age. This is extremely rare, as the group has put years of effort into their training. In generational families, it is almost never a case of "letting someone go." But sometimes they are given false or shielded memories, especially if they are in therapy, to confuse the survivor and the therapist.

The client will need to listen to and believe the internal parties who have more information than he or she does, and take appropriate steps to get to safety. At this point, the client will likely have to cease all contact with the perpetrators. Again, external accountability is paramount. Shelters, women's shelters or church families may be alternatives. One of the worst things the victim can do is to isolate herself, walk alone late at night or go camping alone in the woods. Abduction often occurs in these scenarios, when the survivor is alone and vulnerable. Safe roommates can help keep the survivor safe.

Locking the phone in the trunk of the car can be useful if phone programming is intense. This allows the survivor to wake up or stop phone calls, if an alter has to get up, find the car keys, turn on the light, get out, open the trunk of the car, bring the phone back in and plug it back in before making a phone call.

Establishing a support system through safe support groups, a good therapist, church or work can also be helpful. When possible and practical, moving away from the city or state where the survivor was active in the cult can be helpful. Why? Remember that the survivor's entire support network was the cult in his or her former city. Trainers and/or family members have invested time and effort in the survivor and have a vested interest in the survivor returning. If the survivor moves far enough away, the cult group in his or her new city or state will not know him or her as well and will not have a long history with him or her. This can help reduce the risk of re-accession to the cult, in conjunction with good therapy and a secure support network.

The survivor will have to rebuild his or her support system anyway, so why not do it as far away as possible from the people he or she has known who might hurt him or her? For the survivor, seeing their former coach walking down the street toward them can be an intense trigger, and their inner doubles may be destabilized or feel unsafe. This is a case where distance is a good thing.

Be careful, though: even if the survivor moves, he or she will have to work intensely on blocking the internal recontact programming at the same time, or risk being quickly reconnected. Trainers often send the person's system codes and grids over the Internet to cult groups in the new city, and try to send someone who physically resembles the trainer or a family member to make contact with the survivor.

Internal communication and letting internal alters know they can switch jobs will help. Reward internal reporters who switch allegiances and commit to the survivor's safety. The cult used to reward them for doing their job; now the survivor can reward them for changing jobs. Develop new interests, work, or hobbies that can help the survivor meet new safe people. The survivor may want to practice friendship skills in support groups, as long as they are led by reputable and safe therapists.

Be aware that holidays are often important dates for re-access. There are calendars available showing important holidays for ars groups. Birthdays are also dates when the person is expected to return and there may be programs for this.

Reminder programs (where the person is given a specific date or holiday when they must return to the cult, or be punished) may also need to be stopped. Allowing alters who have been subjected to this programming to share their memories, recognizing their needs, and trying to meet those needs in a healthy way are all healing factors.

The survivor will have to go through a period of grieving for the loss of contact with family members and friends from the cult. Whatever the abuse and dislike, it can be very difficult to break up with the perpetrators, especially if they were the only people close to the survivor. The survivor must recognize the difficulty of creating a new, healthy, non-cult support group. He or she must recognize that learning new skills and developing healthy friendships will take time.

A question often raised by survivors is: How much should I tell others about my past? This is an individual decision that the survivor and therapist need to consider together. In general, it is best to be cautious, because if the survivor tells too much about his or her past, he or she may attract the wrong people to him or her.

These people may be dysfunctional or cult members. It is generally best to base new noncult friendships on the healthy aspects of the person at first and very gradually share small pieces of information as the friendship progresses and sharing seems appropriate. With time and opportunity, the survivor will learn the importance of appropriate boundaries and will want to have healthier relationships in their life.

CHAPTER THIRTEEN

Shell programming, internal guidance, human experimentation, function codes

Some parts of this chapter may be extremely shocking, please read with caution and only with a therapist if you are a survivor. Shell programming is a form of programming used to create a "shell" on the outside, through which other alters on the inside express themselves. It is designed to hide the multiplicity of the person from the outside world and works very well with highly fragmented systems. It also requires a person capable of dissociating to a high degree.

How it happens: in shell programming, the trainer often takes a clear plastic or glass mask and places it in front of the subject. The subject will be extremely traumatized, shocked, drugged, and told that they (the alter(s) in front) are the "mask" that they see. Their job will be to be a shell, or a voice, to cover the others behind. These parts will be so traumatized that they will literally see themselves as a shell, without real substance or body.

The others inside will then be invited to approach the alters in the "shell" and use their voices to cover their own. This allows for more fragmentation of the person, while still being able to hide them from the outside eye, as the inside alters will learn to present themselves through the shell. The alters in the shell always see themselves as "clear" and are not color-coded if color-coded in other systems.

Suggestions

It is important to understand that what the system is actually doing is co-presentation, even if it is not conscious. For a shell program to work, the alters in the shell have been taught to allow co-presentation with the other alters in the system. The other alters in the back are not always aware of what is going on, and the alters in the front, in particular, are not aware that they are being "screened" for co-presentation.

Recognizing the trauma that occurred and discovering where the shell fragments came from will be helpful. Allowing the shell alters and other alters to recognize that this is how they presented themselves, and why, is an important step. The back alters can then begin to introduce themselves without going through the shell, and the person may seem "more multiple" than they ever were for a while, with youthful accents or voices coming through. What actually happens is that the back presents itself without masking what it is through the shell. Meanwhile, the alters in the shell may decide to regroup, for more strength, and may decide to change jobs. Each system will decide what is best for it.

Internal advice

The survivors of the Illuminati programs will always have some form of hierarchy within them. This is because the cult itself is very hierarchical and places that hierarchy within the individual. What better way to inspire loyalty to a leader than to place the leader inside the person's head? Trainers themselves are very concerned with hierarchy. They know that a system without a hierarchy and without a leader on the inside to run things is a system in chaos. They will not leave the person's system without a leader inside.

Many trainers take on the role of the person, to the detriment of programmers or in-house trainers. This is because they are selfish, but also because they use a well-known phenomenon of human nature: PEOPLE TEND TO INTERIORIZE THEIR abusers. The survivor may be horrified to find in himself a representative of one of his worst offenders, but this is a survival mechanism. One of the principles of human behavior is that people will often punish someone who imitates them less. A brutal Nazi will be less likely to punish another brutal Nazi, but will despise and punish a weak and crying person. The survivor will therefore internalize the brutal Nazi in them to avoid being hurt. The survivor may mimic the accents, mannerisms, and even claim the abuser's life story as his own.

The ultimate form of internalization is the internalization of hierarchical guidance. Through pain, hypnosis, and drugs, the person learns to incorporate a highly dissociated group inside to direct others. These groups are often created from divisions of the core, because the trainers want them to be extremely strong and stable alters in the system.

Triads of three elders may be observed. Decks may have a main

board consisting of three people.

The jewels will have a triad, consisting of a ruby, emerald and diamond in many systems, to rule over the others.

And, of course, one can find an internal "governing council," a "system from above," "ascended masters," a "supreme council," a regional council, a world council, etc. The councils found vary according to the survivors.

These inner groups correspond roughly to the outer groups. Often, at the age of twelve, the child or youth is introduced to these groups in a formal coming-of-age ceremony. This ceremony is considered an honor and involves the child being traumatized and accepting the leadership of the council for the rest of their lives. The child is promised unwavering loyalty. There may be other occasions when the person will be forced to appear before the councils during his or her life, either to be judged, to be tested, to be punished, or to be raised. These councils will be seen as holding the power of life and death, and the child or youth will do anything to gain their favor. The child will internalize them. The trainer will assist in the internalization, using photographs or holographic images of the people to "burn" them. Each member of the group will be given different leadership tasks.

It is not uncommon for the survivor to incorporate one, both or both parents or grandparents into their internal leadership hierarchy in the case of a generational survivor.

High priests and priestesses may serve on the governing councils within. Suggestions:

Internal boards of directors are often among the most resistant and hostile to therapy, especially in the early stages. They verbally banter with the therapist or refuse to talk to him or her, believing that he or she is "beneath them." They mimic the haughty, hierarchical attitudes they have been exposed to all their lives.

They also have the most to lose if the survivor leaves the cult, and may fight this decision tooth and nail. It is often the alters who have an "attitude.

Both the survivor and the therapist need to recognize that these parties had important needs that were met within the cult. Ignoring this and arguing with them will only reinforce their belief that therapists are stupid and ignorant people. Acknowledge their internal role while gently pointing out reality. Try to get their help to help the survivor get stronger. Have an honest discussion about the pros and cons of leaving the cult. These are highly intellectual alters who need to express their concerns and doubts. It is important to set good boundaries and not allow verbal abuse of the therapist. These alters are used to "pushing people around" verbally and have been rewarded for this before therapy. They now need to learn new coping skills and behaviors, and this process may take time. Allow them to express their anger, dissatisfaction and fears about the decision to leave the cult. Offer them new jobs with the person running the safety committees or even the decision-making committees.

Sometimes a system that has broken free from the cult and has no external hierarchy to which it is accountable goes through a short period of chaos when the news spreads: we are free and no longer have to do what the cult tells us to do! Hundreds of internal arguments can break out about what we are going to do for a living, where we are going to live, what we are going to eat, what our hobbies are. Everyone wants to get out, see the day and live this new free life. But freedom can cause an imbalance with all the changes going on inside. Helping the internal hierarchy and creating a limited democracy with ground rules can be helpful during this time. Do not dismantle the internal hierarchy overnight, or systems will be rudderless. Seek their help in steering the survivor in the right direction. Things will calm down after a while, when systems learn to listen to each other, vote on ideas and move together in the same direction.

Human experimentation

This is one of the most serious things that is still going on with the Illuminati today. The Illuminati were famous for deciding years ago to "go scientific" and incorporate scientific experimentation into their training principles. This is an area in which they broke with other more traditional groups, which still followed "spiritual principles. The Illuminati decided to use scientific data, particularly in the psychiatric and behavioral sciences, to guide their training practices. This practice became openly known during World War II, when the world heard about the experiments conducted on Jews and other groups in concentration camps, but the experiments on human beings had been going on quietly for years before going underground.

Nor did it stop when the war ended. German trainers and scientists were scattered around the world and hidden away, where they continued to teach others the principles they had learned and to continue their experiments.

Some of these experiments were funded by the government through groups such as the CIA and NSA. The Illuminati had infiltrators in these groups, who used the principles they discovered and shared them with their own trainers.

The experimentation is still going on today. It is done in secret. Its purpose is to help improve and create more sophisticated training techniques. It is to prevent "programming failures", or "PFS" as they are called in the cult.

Many, if not all, survivors have been told that they were just an experiment. This can be true or false. Trainers like to tell their subjects that they are experiments, even if they are not, for several reasons:

1. It creates immense fear and a feeling of helplessness in the subject (he thinks to himself that if this is an experiment, I will have to work very hard to survive it).

2. This devalues the person enormously. They will feel that they have no real value as a human being, that they are just an experiment. A person who feels devalued doesn't care and will be willing to do things that they wouldn't do if they felt some value, some humanization.

3. This gives the trainer additional power, because he or she can start or stop the "experiment. Almost always, when the person is told that they are an experiment, this is not really the case. When trainers and cult members actually do experiments, the subjects are never told because it could skew the results. Fear could interfere with the effects of the drugs and distort the results. The most recent cult experiments have focused on the effects of drugs: the use of different drugs, both alone and in new combinations and dosages, to induce trance states and open the person to training. Drugs are sought that shorten the time interval needed to induce the trance state, are rapidly metabolized, and leave no detectable residue the next day.

Behavioral science: observing and recording data on various environmental parameters on human behavior. Modifying the environment.

Praise and punishment as motivators

Isolation techniques: recording of physiological and psychological data from different isolation methods. Removal, addition, combination of different sensory isolation methods and the effect of each.

Effectiveness of the virtual reality in the programming of the implementation. Effectiveness of new disks created to incorporate programming. The cult's graphics and computer experts will work to create better and more effective VR disks, which will be tested for effectiveness on cult subjects. The cult wants more and more standardization and less room for human error and weakness in their training techniques, so they are using more and more high-tech equipment and videos. Attempts to break programming, cause program failure, record what works and what doesn't, and develop new sequences to prevent FP. Subjects under hypnosis are instructed to try to break certain internal programming sequences. The ways in which they do this and what appears to be effective are reported to the trainers, who then create new programs to prevent programming breakdown.

Harmony/light, sensory deprivation and overstimulation and their neurological and physical effects. New combinations of sensory input are constantly being tested to determine which ones give the most lasting results and can be achieved quickly.

The cult is always trying to find new, better and faster ways to break down subjects, introduce programming and prevent programming from failing.

This is the result of much of the research she has conducted. The results of this research are shared around the world, both through the Internet, phone calls and international trainers' conferences, where trainers from around the world share their research findings. New techniques are incorporated by other groups eager to learn what is discovered.

Suggestions

If you have experimental programming, be aware that the alters who have been used are very traumatized. They feel devalued, less than human, and this has been strongly reinforced by the trainers who have worked with them. They were probably not used in the initial experiments, as described above, but may have been used in second-level experiments.

I will explain what these terms mean.

The best trainers and leaders will launch an experiment with a new drug. They will learn to fiddle with the dosages and record all the observable facts on hundreds of subjects. When they have collected enough data, they will allow it to be used by trainers in local groups. The experiment will then still be considered experimental, but it will be second-tier, not first-tier. At this point, all trainers in the local groups will be asked to record and report any adverse drug reactions, usual dosages needed, etc. This data is collected in data banks (yes, the cult has entered the computer age), inside encrypted files, which will then be sent to a central base in Langley, Virginia.

The alters used in experiments, or who have been told they are experiments, need to understand that they have value. They need to realize that they have been subjected to intense programming and be allowed to express themselves and discuss their experiences. The fear associated with the belief that they are an experiment must be appropriately vented. They will be angry at the dehumanization, intentionality, and coldness of what they have experienced, and rightly so. They may resent the effects in their current lives of the experiences and procedures they underwent, and need to grieve the loss of body image, the loss of trust in people, the sense of betrayal and powerlessness they felt during the procedures. They may want to keep a journal or make drawings of their experiences.

A warm, empathetic therapist who listens, believes, and does not minimize what they have experienced is invaluable at this point. Allowing the internal cognitives and helpers to anchor the parts that have been having bizarre sensory experiences, and creating "anchor committees" internally will also help. Additional support may be needed to cope with such intense experiences and feelings.

Function codes

Trainers place in the subject's systems a special way of organizing the fragments related to the work for which they have been trained. These codes are called function codes and there are three main types:

Command codes: these are irreversible commands, introduced at the limbic level of conditioning. The first code always introduced is the "stop" command, which stops the person in his tracks, and it is the first code that any new trainer learns. It prevents the subject from murdering his trainer, if he has undergone MK ULTRA or other murder training.

Other command codes include: system destruction (suicide)

codes, burst codes, erase codes and anti-suicide codes.

Access codes: These are specialized codes, often coded as short messages or numeric codes, that allow access to the person's system. A trainer will always begin a session by repeating the person's full personal access code, which will allow them to enter the system without triggering internal traps and protections. These codes may also depend on the visual and voice recognition of the person giving them. In other words, the system will only respond to codes if someone who appears to be an authorized person, such as the person's trainer, gives them. This is to prevent unauthorized access or use of the person by others outside the local cult group.

Function Codes: These are the "job codes" or work codes within the system. Often several of these are coded to be linked together to perform a task. It is usually a letter, such as a letter of the Greek alphabet, combined with a numerical sequence that corresponds to their place on the internal grid or landscape.

Suggestions

If the survivor has function codes or other internal codes, it will be helpful if the various controllers in the system share them with the person. The person can then get to know the fragments, hear their history, and help them begin to coalesce with other internal parts. It may be helpful to find the model from which these codes were fragmented and to help the model realize how it was traumatized to create these fragments.

About deprogrammers: Often people who call themselves deprogrammers try to find these codes and help the person. This is an individual decision of each survivor and therapist. There can be excellent deprogrammers, but I have always been extremely cautious and have never used one for two reasons:

1. I will never again relinquish the locus of control to an outside person. It would be too much of a reminder of the abuse I suffered, and I think the survivor needs to take charge of themselves in therapy as much as possible.

2. There are no quick fixes, miracles or shortcuts in the process of undoing the many abuses that have been committed in Illuminati programming. Even the best deprogrammers admit that once they are done, the person usually has an idea of what was put

into them, but that they need to finish with years of therapy to find out how they feel about the programming that was done. A realistic therapist will realize that it will take years of patience, support, and hard work on the part of the therapist and the survivor to undo a lifetime of conditioning and pain. This is not to say that deprogrammers don't help people; good, reputable and safe deprogrammers have been reported to be of great help. But the person can also undertake the process of undoing their own programming, and often the survivor is the best "internal deprogrammer" of all. They know better than anyone else the people inside them and what motivates them.

CHAPTER FOURTEEN

Spiritual programming

Note: this chapter deals with both the spirituality of cults and Christian spirituality; do not read it if these topics bother you.

* * *

Any discussion of Illuminati programming would be incomplete without addressing spiritual programming. Most of the previous chapters have dealt with scientific, organized and structured programming.

But the Illuminati are not primarily scientists, but spiritualists. The very foundation of the group is based on the occult. And they go to great lengths to integrate these occult beliefs into the systems of their people.

The importance of spiritual programming in a person's systems varies from person to person and depends on the individual group, their religious heritage, the beliefs of the leader and the group's trainers.

All children participate in rituals, where they are consecrated from before birth and at regular intervals throughout their lives. During these rituals, demonic entities are invoked to force the person into servitude, loyalty, and secrecy, as well as to reinforce ongoing programming.

Trainers will invoke the demonic overlay during programming sessions. This is done after an acute trauma. The person is asked if they want to suffer more, and they will always say "no". The trainer then offers a solution: if they accept one or more "protectors", they will not suffer anymore. Trainers want this because they know that with these "protectors" they can shorten the training sessions. The protectors, or guardians, will reinforce the programming internally, without outside help. This concept will seem controversial to those who do not believe in spiritual realities, but I am merely describing what the enlightened believe and what their trainers practice.

Spiritual programming will also include the requirement to memorize rituals, the BOOK OF ILLUMINATION and other books containing cult beliefs. The person will be saturated with cult beliefs from childhood, in classes and training sessions. He or she will attend rituals in which adults participate in spiritual cults, wear robes and prostrate themselves before the group's tutelary deity. Moloch, Ashtaroth, Baal, Enokkim are commonly worshipped demons. The child may witness a sacrifice, real or simulated, to these deities; animal sacrifices are common. The child will be forced to participate in the sacrifices and will have to go through blood baptism.

They will be forced to remove the heart or other internal organs from a sacrificial animal and eat them. The adults and leaders of the group place their hands on the head of the child, who is drugged, and summon demonic entities.

One of the rituals that is actually scheduled is the "resuscitation ritual". During this ritual, the child may be heavily drugged and shocked or tortured to the point that his heart stops. The head priest then "resuscitates" the child, using drugs, cardiopulmonary resuscitation and incantations. When the child comes to and is awake, he is told that he has been "brought back to life" by the demonic entity that the group worships, and that the child now owes him his life. He is told that if he says so or tries to make the demon go away, he will return to the inanimate state he was in before the reanimation.

Spiritual "healings" from the demon are also common. Wounds caused by torture, programming sessions or even military exercises will be healed almost instantly during invocations.

Jewelry programming often includes demons loyal to generational family spirits. These are called "family jewels". The demons "guard" them and help protect the programming around them.

In a sense, every ritual a young child participates in is an intense programming experience, as the child observes the adults around him or her and imitates their behavior. The child will be severely punished if he or she falls asleep and will be told that the demons will kill him or her if he or she falls asleep again during a ritual.

They are taught to remain completely silent no matter what they see during the rituals. The child will witness things that seem quite unbelievable, including faces transformed by demons, channeling, other voices coming out of a leader's mouth, reading members, predicting the future. Members who can channel powerful spirits and survive are respected and their advice is sought after.

Some groups will use scripture in a negative way or program the child to hate Christian symbols and theology. Other groups will encourage the amnesiac front to adopt a Christian lifestyle, while forcing the former altars to deny and blaspheme the choices made by the front, in order to further separate the two groups of altars. The alters of the sect will be told that since they have renounced Christianity, they have committed the "unpardonable sin" and can never be forgiven. They will be shown biblical texts that are supposed to support this claim.

In moments of despair, during intense torture or isolation, a person often calls on God for help. Trainers or other cult members often mock the person by telling them that God has forgotten them or asking, "Where is God now? He must hate you..."

Any negative experience the person has will be used to reinforce the idea that they have been abandoned by God. The cult will happily point out the contradictions between what the person is experiencing and what Christianity teaches should happen to them.

They may distort scriptures or use false scriptures. They can distort Christian hymns or use them in programming. One of the favorite hymns is "Let the circle be unbroken" because it can have two meanings.

Suggestions

Spiritual programming can be one of the most damaging in a person's system, as it attempts to cut them off from the source of true healing. It is an intentional distortion of the truth, with events calculated to teach and reinforce erroneous concepts of God. Many survivors are unable to hear Christian terms or are intensely offended by any religious discussion.

The survivor and therapist must understand that these negative reactions are the result of years of misguided teaching, pain, punishment, distortion and entrapment. It is important not to judge the parts of the person that are negative about spirituality, or that express themselves by proclaiming the power and benefits of cult spirituality.

The survivor's front may be horrified to hear or learn that some parts are experiencing these feelings, especially if they are a committed Christian. These inner parts share the only reality they have ever known and need time and patience to take root and experience reality outside the cult setting.

It may be necessary to treat demonic oppression, even deliverance, to relieve a system terrorized by the demon.

Each therapist and survivor will have to accept their own spiritual beliefs. Personally, I think a therapist should consider the possibility of the demonic, since that is what the survivor has been exposed to his or her entire life. The cult certainly believes it is real, and anyone who has been involved in a cult setting has had experiences that cannot be explained by normal rational scientific principles.

The survivor needs hope and healing. A positive spirituality based on love, gentleness, and forgiveness, as opposed to the coercive, punitive, and negative spirituality that the survivor has experienced, will greatly assist in the healing process. A spiritual belief system that offers hope, healing, grace, mercy, and affirmation will often provide the survivor with the support they need to continue the often difficult healing process.

CHAPTER FIFTEEN

Trunk splits, negation programming, the last five steps of the discipline

Virtual reality programming

Virtual reality (VR) programming is a form of programming that has come into widespread use over the past few decades. It involves the person being placed in a virtual reality headset and suit while a virtual reality disc created by an artist is used to run the program. It can be used to create 3D and holographic images, and is particularly useful for script programming and target practice sequences for assassin training. Under hypnosis, the person will actually believe they are in the scene.

Virtually any scenario can be recreated. The images to be "burned" will be displayed on the VR disk and reinforced repeatedly during the programming sequence. Some trainers believe that this eliminates the "human error" element in training and use it quite extensively. VR programming, like any other programming, involves going inside and discovering the distortions that have been placed in the parts that have been programmed, allowing them to see how they have been deceived, and dealing with the trauma associated with the programming.

The programming of denial

Denial programming begins with the infant's first experiences. The child has been horribly injured and traumatized, but the next morning, the adults around the child act normally, as if nothing had happened. They model for the infant and toddler a lifestyle of denial. This attitude is reinforced later by telling the child:

"It was just a bad dream" (oh, how the child wants to believe this lie. It eases the pain of thinking it didn't really happen) "it's just your imagination, it didn't really happen" (which is again accepted as an escape from the horror). Denial is also fueled by the adults around the child, who tell them that they will never be believed if they reveal it.

Devices will be put in place to teach the child what they see and hear, and to teach them to trust outside adults to tell them their reality.

A typical installation is as follows:

The adult holds an object, such as an orange, in his or her hand and asks the young child, aged two or three, "What is this? The child will quickly respond, "Oh, an orange! The child will be shocked and told, "No, it's an apple. The child will be confused, because what he or she is looking at is obviously an orange. It's the color orange, it smells like orange, it looks like an orange. The question will be repeated. The child may answer "an orange" again and be shocked again. Finally, the child, unsure and not wanting to be punished, will say "an apple" and be praised.

The purpose of this exercise is to teach the child not to trust their own reality and to look to outside adults or leaders to tell them what reality really is.

This is the basis of denial: the person learns not to trust their own reality, because of the punishment and fear they feel when they have told the truth.

Alters will be created as the child grows up, whose purpose is to deny the cult's abuse. In the event of an escape or breakthrough, the job of the denial alters is to create a plausible explanation: it was a nightmare, a book the person read, a movie they saw, etc. These alters will read and cite literature that refutes RSA. THESE ALTERS OFTEN BELIEVE THAT THEY ARE SAVING THE SURVIVOR'S LIFE.

They were told that if the survivor remembered and believed in the abuse, he or she would be killed, or that the denial alter would be severely punished or broken for not doing their job. These parties have a vested interest in their work: they believe that their very existence and the survival of their body depends on them.

Suggestions

Arguing with a person in denial will not work because they are not motivated by logic, but by fear. A better approach is to ask them what they fear if they remember. This will open the door to deception and lies that have been ingrained. They may be protecting the survivor from suicidal alters who are behind them and are programmed to intervene if the denial is broken. It is helpful to allow them to express their concerns and to call on helpers or cognates who do not have a suicidal or denial agenda. Showing them reality in a gentle way, allowing them to "listen" to others who share the same thing is a big step forward.

Some denials are the natural consequence of self-protection against the horrors of abuse; not all denials are programmatic. But if denial consistently blocks therapy and paralyzes it completely, if the person becomes very suicidal every time denial is briefly set aside, this possibility should be considered. Safety, inner cooperation and patience will go a long way to reducing denial. When denial recedes, immense grief work is to be expected as the truth emerges. Denial has protected the survivor from the horrible pain of the truth and must be let go very slowly and carefully, with much support during the grieving phase.

Splitting of the core

Basic splits are intentional traumatic splits created from the basic personality.

The core can literally be "split" by overwhelming psychological and physical/spiritual trauma. The trauma necessary to create a split in the nucleus must be very early and psychologically devastating. Fetal splits can occur, but it is rarely a core split; instead, the core creates an alteration, but remains.

Core separation occurs between the ages of 18 months and 3 years. Usually at least one parent or primary caregiver is involved in the trauma, as this creates the psychological devastation necessary for core separation. Physical trauma alone rarely causes the core to crack. The torture is intense and prolonged, until the child collapses. It may involve shocks, stretching, hanging from a height, or a combination of techniques. Placement in "shock boxes" or near-drowning are also used.

Techniques that create core splits are also dangerous, as they can also cause autism if the child cannot handle the programming. When I was in the cult, I fought to stop core splitting because sometimes children were lost or the founding personality was too weakened.

The nucleus can divide into two, three or up to eight internal parts. Each division will be a piece of the "child nucleus". The original core will not resurface after the split. These splits are used by cult trainers as models for creating systems within the child. A split from the core, or a split from a core, will be a strong alter, and can be split several times in the programming process, to create a multifaceted and diverse system within the child.

Suggestions

Core splits represent an intense founding trauma. They form the basis for later systems, which can be completely dissociated from the split over time. Work on core splits should be done very slowly, and only at the end of the therapy process, when there is immense cooperation within the system. The survivor will need all of his or her internal resources to cope with these traumas, as well as significant external therapeutic support.

This may mean hospitalization, unless the survivor is able to keep the trauma from emerging too quickly, and the therapist and survivor go extremely slowly.

Other less disjointed systems and fragments should be integrated.

Cognitive recognition of the abuse will be the first step in processing the core trauma. Allowing the more dissociated parts to grieve by "hearing about" what happened can come next. Allowing the feelings close to the core to come together, little by little, with the help of supportive internal helpers and nannies can be helpful.

These feelings need to be measured out and explored bit by bit. Children may be of different ages and need to express themselves in different ways.

There may be "dream programming", a "fantasy world" or some other form of escape from reality surrounding the divided core, which protects them from contact with the outside world, perceived as brutal and cold.

Some parts can be completely disconnected from the external reality in order to reduce the pain.

Slow, patient care and reality orientation will help these terribly traumatized parts begin to reach the outer reality. Some parts will have always been aware of what happened, but will not care to rejoin the outside world.

Patience, allowing them to express themselves, is most helpful.

Stages of Discipline: Step Seven: Don't Worry About It

This stage will take him further into an aggressive role. He will be forced to hurt others and prove his ability to care less about others in the process.

Eighth step: time travel

The child will be taught the spiritual principles of the inner and outer "journey" with dramatization, role-playing and guided exercises reinforced by trauma. The goal is to achieve "Enlightenment," an ecstatic state of dissociation achieved after severe trauma.

Steps nine, ten, eleven

This will be a program that will vary depending on the child's future role in the cult. Sexual trauma, learning to disassociate and increase cognition, decrease feelings will be emphasized in these stages.

Stage Twelve: "The Transition to Adulthood"

A coming-of-age ceremony at the age of twelve or thirteen, where the child is formally inducted into the cult and his or her adult role in a coming-of-age ceremony. He or she will prove his or her ability to perform the role/job for which he or she has been trained, to the satisfaction of the trainer and leaders, by undergoing a special induction ceremony. The ritual and ceremony takes place with other children of the same age, who are dressed in white and receive an award in recognition of successfully completing the basics of their training.

They will continue to be abused, even into adulthood, but the major trauma and system patterning will have taken place at this age. Future training will refine what has already been put in place in the child at this age, or build on the foundation.

Suggestions

It is important to grieve the abuse and acknowledge the feelings associated with the trauma. It will be necessary to address the issue of perpetrator guilt, as by this time the child will be a perpetrator and will have identified with the adult role models around them. This can be difficult, as the perpetration of the act horrifies the survivor when they remember it. It is important to support the survivor, be non-judgmental and encourage acceptance of these parts. Pointing out that at the time there were no other options available can be helpful. The realization that the perpetrator's alters saved the child's life and had no other way to act, especially initially, the first time, should be stressed. The survivor may feel hostile or vilified by the perpetrator's doubles, but they are an expression of the abuse and limited choices left to them. Grieving from an abuser will take time and will require the caring support of others.

TESTIMONY OF SVALI, FORMER ILLUMINATI

Centrexnews.com article series. Published with permission of the U.S. Publisher. Source:
www.educate-yourself.org/mcsvaliinterviewpt1.html

This article is part of a series of articles that are transcripts of a series of exclusive interviews conducted by centrexnews' Senior Editor, HJ Springer. He asked Svali a number of specific questions via email regarding the Illuminati in America and around the world. Svali is a woman who has held significant training responsibilities within the Illuminati group. After her conversion to Jesus Christ, she decided to testify, while wishing to remain anonymous.

Note from the Editor of educate-yourself.org, who released this series of interviews:

It was Brice Taylor who brought this series of interviews to my attention. They confirm in an excellent way the behavior and nature of the Illuminati "families" that Brice Taylor talks about in his book "Thanks for the Memories". But it also offers an interesting addition, concerning the work of a programmer in the field of mind control. The latter's work is more "clinical" (though abominable). This work is just as destructive to the victims of such mind control as it is to the programmers themselves, who are most of the time under the influence of that same mind control. Neither of them are aware that they are involved in such a destructive activity. All of them, however, are directly involved in this diabolical program of enslavement, the genesis of which goes back to the Nazi concentration camps, under the direction of Dr. Joseph Mengele, the infamous "angel of death" of

Auschwitz. It was this same Dr. Joseph Mengele who finished developing this program, right here in the United States, thanks to the OSS/CIA and the "Paper Clip" operation.

H. J. Springer, Editor of centrexnews.com, has written some introductory remarks to his series of interviews with Svali. We are grateful to "Svali" for revealing this information, and to H. J. Springer for writing these articles. You can read more of Svali's articles and his book of testimonies on his website www.suite101.com. All thinking people on our planet should be aware of the Illuminati power agenda. Otherwise, their lives, and the lives of their children, will have to bear the terrible consequences of their negligence, ignorance, and inaction.

Introduction by H. J. Springer, senior editor of centrexnews.com:

When we ran our series of articles on "How the Illuminati Program People," we received a number of rather skeptical emails asking for more information. Needless to say, I had a number of questions myself about the Illuminati and their agenda. So I contacted Svali (that's a pseudonym), a former Illuminati programmer and trainer, to ask her about her testimony. I have done my best to ensure that the following articles will enlighten you (pardon the pun), and give you the additional information I was able to receive from Svali.

Our correspondence took the form of an interview by e-mail. I hardly edited them at all. I only edited the spelling and punctuation, and removed some personal information about myself. I'll now move on to the first part of our interviews.

FIRST PART

Svali introduces himself

Dear Mr. Springler,

Thank you for contacting me. I have to tell you that I just received a rather skeptical e-mail today from someone who has been looking at your site. I would be very happy to answer your questions, but with the following caveat. I am writing under a pseudonym, to protect my two children and my husband. I don't want them to receive hostile phone calls or threats or anything like that. Both of my children are still healing from the experiences of being raised in this group. I don't want them to have any more traumatic experiences.

The topic I am about to address is a delicate one, to say the least. People often have strong reactions, positive or negative, when they want to know if the Illuminati really exist. That said, I'm going to tell you a little about myself. Then you are free to see if you can share this information with your readers. I also write regularly on the subject of ritual abuse, at http://www.suite101.com. You can also do a search on "Svali". I have written a number of articles on this topic, in case you want to know more.

I was born in 1957 in Alexandria, Virginia, USA. I lived for a short time in a small town about an hour's drive from Washington, D.C. Then we moved to a 200-acre farm in northern Virginia, where my mother married my stepfather. My stepfather and mother were part of the Illuminati. It's a group where you're Illuminati from generation to generation. My mother was on the Regional Council for the Washington, D.C. area. The Illuminati have six chairs in their councils. These chairs correspond to the areas of focus of their "Perfected Masters. These six chairs are in the following areas: Science, Government, High Leaders, Education, Spiritual Domain, and Military Domain.

These are also the areas in which the children of cult members are trained. They believe that they must have "well-trained" children. The "spiritual" education was only a small part of what was taught in this group, as the training was also extensive in the other five areas. I spent more time learning history, modern languages, and science than undergoing occult rituals, although the latter were very important to the group.

I attended school in Charlottesville, Virginia from 1975 to 1981. I am a registered nurse, and I also have an undergraduate degree in Spanish. It is a facility where a lot of abuse and occult crimes are practiced. It is located on an estate about 18 miles southwest of Charlottesville, going towards Crowley, Virginia.

After graduating with both degrees, I went to San Diego, California in 1981. I was called there by the local leaders of the group. They were very strong in military education, but weak in science, which was my forte. I was accepted to serve on the leadership council. I was the sixth trainer in order of preeminence, which was the last of the senior trainers. I had 30 trainers under me, spread out in the local groups. The leadership council met in Ramona at a property owned by a man named Jonathan Meiers... One of his occult code names was "Black Hand," because he used to wear black gloves when he worked with people. He was the chief trainer of this group, and one of the most brutal and sadistic men I have ever known. He completely wore down almost every trainer who worked with him, except me, because I had a friend on the leadership council who hated him and helped me undermine his authority. The Illuminati are very political, and they love to backstab each other. They fight like dogs, because everyone wants to climb higher. My friend's secret name was Athena.

After twelve years of working with Jonathan, I was promoted to the position of second lead trainer for the county. Jonathan was preparing to move up to the regional level, and he wanted me to take his place. But we despised each other, and he set a trap for me to fall. That's a whole other story, but it was one of the factors that made me leave that group. I left the group in 1995, fed up with all the lies, deceit, and dirty tricks. I also feared for my life. I fled to Texas and underwent therapy with Dr. Jerry Mundgaze and his group. Unfortunately, they did not know how to "deprogram" me. As Dr. Mundgaze said to me, "You are on a much higher level than almost anyone we have ever known, and you are much more deeply programmed.

I remembered a lot of things, things he had never heard, and he didn't know how to help me. Most of my memories came back to me spontaneously, at home. I was never hypnotized to allow me to dig into my memories. They came back to me in the course of my normal daytime activities.

I spent a whole year intensively deprogramming myself. Since I was the head programmer, I was able to use what I knew to undo all the programming I had gone through. I was in a rage, realizing that all the abuse I had to go through, and that I had put others through, was not something normal, but had been used to manipulate me.

The book I wrote to give my testimony is based on my memories as an adult in the Illuminati group. I did some criminal things, and now I deeply regret it. My way of making restitution, before God, is to expose the doctrines and practices of this group. I also wrote this book to help therapists understand the methods of this group. Because it was quite common to hear ritual abuse centers say, "We don't know what to do..." I used what I was able to put into practice myself to get my healing.

Two years ago, my children, who were visiting my home, told me about the abuse they had suffered at the hands of their father. I went to the social services, but my case was dismissed because the official in charge told me that she did not believe in the reality of ritual abuse! When my ex-husband came to claim the children, he could have put me in jail for not returning the children. The San Diego court had coldly declared that he did not believe in the reality of ritual abuse. In all cases of ritual abuse, the children are given to the parent who was accused of doing the abuse!

My children did not hesitate to confront their father directly. He turned white as a sheet and said, "So you really don't want to go back to the 'family'?" They said, "No!" He flew back to California, quit his job, and moved here. He agreed to go to therapy, for various personality disorders. My children are also in therapy and are healing quickly. My son, who is 12 now, is almost completely recovered and happier than ever. My daughter, who is sixteen, has some difficult issues to deal with because she was sexually abused. But God has been faithful, and we see that he is healing all of us.

I wish that everything we experienced had not really happened. But it did. We are getting a lot of confirmed testimonies about everything that is going on in this area, especially about ritual abuse. I could send you those testimonies. My biggest regret is that I was used by this group, after a whole career as a trainer, to perpetrate the most criminal acts. I have often tortured and abused people who I thought I was "helping" by these means!

I realize now that I was wrong. I have asked God to forgive me. And I am determined to expose what the Illuminati are doing through the written word. Professionally, I also write articles in the medical field, having worked as a registered nurse for over 18 years. I also now work as a trainer in the health field.

I hope that this is enough for you as a personal testimony. Before God and men, I speak the truth. If you want to know more, without jeopardizing my anonymity or the protection of my children, please let me know.

Sincerely,

P.S. My youngest sister remembers being gagged and tied to a stone altar at the age of three to be raped. She also remembers our paternal grandmother taking her to friends for sexual abuse between the ages of 3 and 5. She became an alcoholic at 13, and had committed 7 suicide attempts by the age of 12. One of my brothers, who is older than I am, has absolutely no memory of anything that happened to him before he was 20 years old. His whole past is like a black hole. He believes, however, that our father was a strange and perverse man. This brother had tried to hang himself in our garage when he was 8 years old.

My older brother is always moving. He is afraid to stay in one place for more than a few months because he thinks "they want to get him". He too has tried to commit suicide many times as a child.

These are just a few more proofs of what is going on in this group. I could also cite the fact that my two children dream in German. This is the language they use between Illuminati. Yet they have never heard this language spoken!

SECOND PART

Who are the Illuminati?

Question: *Are you embarrassed to testify on this subject?*

Svali's answer: I don't mind talking about the Illuminati. I simply explained why I was using a pseudonym. I recently received a letter saying that I was using a pseudonym because I was a fraud, which is not true at all. Because I write articles in medical magazines on health topics, I know that it is important to cite facts that can be verified. That's why I didn't mind at all that you wanted to hear my story. In fact, it shows me that you are a responsible editor, which I admire. I have nothing to hide. My story is one hundred percent true.

I have not gained anything financially by giving my testimony. I refuse to perform on television. I am unknown, and I prefer to remain unknown. I don't get any royalties from doing what I do. I just want to pay my children's medical bills. That means I have three part-time jobs! This is to answer the skeptics who say that people testify to gain sympathy from others. I am not looking for sympathy and I don't need it. I have made choices in my life, and I have made mistakes, but I am now working to make restitution. While I'm on the subject of money, I will say that I make $20 a month for my work on my Suite 101 site. I make $150 to $250 for every article I write on women's health. Guess what topics I write about most often. Women's health! And not at all on the topic of ritual abuse! The editors of the health magazines that publish my articles have absolutely no idea of the topics I write about. This is also why I write under a pseudonym. I don't write to become famous. On the contrary, if my colleagues knew about my past, I would risk losing my job! I have everything to lose by exposing the Illuminati, and everything to gain by remaining silent.

But I also know that ritual abuse of children must be stopped. As a Christian, and as an activist against ritual child abuse, I have decided to bear witness to this abuse by the Illuminati, by writing articles against it. I also know that many very qualified people have already published their testimony on this subject. They might be an interesting additional resource for you. But I don't know any of them personally, as I have no contact with any cult survivors outside of my own family. However, it is a possibility.

Let's get to your questions.

Question: Svali, I think our readers are wondering if the Illuminati are members of a religion or a secret society, if they are involved in Satanism, or if they combine all these activities. Is it something different again, or more sinister?

Answer: The Illuminati are followers of a doctrine called "Enlightenment". They are a Luciferian group that teaches their followers that their roots are in the ancient mysteries of Babylon, Egypt, and the Celtic druids. They claim to have retained the "best" of these esoteric traditions, integrating them with a strong occult discipline. Locally, many Illuminati groups worship ancient gods such as El, Baal, Astarte, Isis, Osiris, and Set.

That said, the leadership council members sometimes scoff at the more "primitive" practices that occur at lower levels of the hierarchy. When I was on the San Diego council, I remember them calling the high priests and high priestesses "public entertainers" who spent their time "distracting the base." I don't mean to offend anyone, but simply to show that the leaders are convinced that they are driven by more scientific and intellectual criteria. But they all practice the principles of "enlightenment".

Enlightenment consists of twelve steps, also known as the "twelve steps of discipline. It also includes learning astral travel, time travel, and other occult powers. Are these abilities real, or are they drug-induced hallucinations? I can't say. I have witnessed things that cannot be explained rationally, things that have frightened me. But, all I can say is that it could be a combination of mind control, drug influence, and true demonic activity. In what proportion? I don't know. But I do know that these people are teaching and practicing evil.

At the highest levels of the Illuminati, it is no longer a matter of people in black robes making incantations around a big fire. The boards of directors include administrators who handle the finances. Believe me, they make a lot of money. If that were the only reason, it would be enough to keep these groups going, let alone all the religious filth that goes on. The leaders of the Illuminati include bankers, businessmen, and city and political leaders. They are intelligent, well-educated, and active in their churches. Above the local governing councils are the regional councils, which control the local groups. They help set policy and programs at the regional level and manage the activity of the local councils.

At the national level, there are extremely wealthy people who finance the activities of the cult and who have connections with the leaders of other countries. The Illuminati is an international group. All their activities are covered by absolute secrecy. The first thing a child must learn about the "family," or "Order," as they still call it, is the need for secrecy. That's why you don't hear much from the survivors who made it through. The members of this group have a very long arm and know what to do to terrify those who would like to be a little too talkative. The children are taught not to talk, by terrorizing them with macabre scenes. The children are then told that those who suffered these horrible fates (sometimes fabricated for "educational" purposes) are traitors who had to be punished. The vision of these terrible scenes remains imprinted for life in the memory of these young children of 3 or 4 years. When they become adults, even when they manage to leave the group, many of them are not encouraged to speak out for fear of being found and punished.

I myself have participated in many of these macabre productions, as a trainer. So I have become somewhat cynical, which is why I chose to speak. However, I still experience very intense scares from time to time. Imagine the reactions of a four year old locked in a wooden box for a while and then buried in a hole! Even if he only stays there for a few minutes, those minutes are worth an eternity to that child! Then, when he is released, he is told, "If you ever talk, we'll put you back in there, and this time we'll leave you there!" That child will start screaming hysterically that he will never tell! This is what I have experienced personally. Now I have decided to break this law of silence, which was imposed on me by these psychological tortures. Because I don't want other children to know what I experienced and what I saw practiced.

Yes, the Illuminati are well organized, very secretive, and extremely wealthy at the highest levels. They are not stupid. They are not poor people who play at witchcraft. You are very much mistaken if you see them that way.

Question: *What is the extent of the Illuminati's infiltration of society? Are there many of them? Are they present in every city in the United States? Are they recruiting people who are not members of their group?*

How far do the members of this group go to keep this knowledge secret?

Answer: I think I have already answered your question about secrecy. The Illuminati are present in every major city in the United States. They have divided the United States into 7 major regions, each under the authority of a regional council that controls all the local councils in their district. They meet every two months, and on special occasions.

A region may have from 10 to 30 local groups. In rural areas, members meet with the nearest local groups under the direction of their regional council. They almost never recruit people who are not members of their sect. However, they sometimes buy children from Asian families, for example, and keep them under their constant supervision. In exchange, they protect them from the actions of local mafias. They are threatened to hand them over to the mafias if they talk.

The Illuminati also have excellent lawyers who are paid handsomely to cover up all their activities. They also pay people who work in the media to keep stories out of the papers. I know of three people in San Diego who worked for the Union Tribune (a local newspaper) who were Illuminati loyalists. They often wrote articles attacking local doctors who were trying to treat survivors of ritual abuse. I remember hearing some of our governing council members bragging about how they had driven One Tel out of town because of a media campaign, and how proud they were of it.

The Illuminati believe they can control a region, if they can control :

➢ Banks and financial institutions. You'd be surprised how many Illuminati sit on the boards of these organizations!

➢ Local authorities. You'd also be surprised how many Illuminati get elected to city councils!

➢ Legal institutions, as well as law and medical schools. Children in the cult are encouraged to study law and medicine.

➢ Media. Children are also encouraged to study journalism. Some Illuminati also fund the creation of local newspapers.

Question: *Are the Illuminati the same as those created by Adam Weishaupt in Germany?*

Answer: It was not Weishaupt who created the Illuminati. They simply chose him as a figurehead and told him what to write. It was financiers who created the Illuminati, back in the days of the Templar Order.

These men financed kings all over Europe. Weishaupt was only their front man, who obeyed the orders he received.

Question: *Do you have any other information about the political goals of the Illuminati, if they have any?*

Answer: I wrote an article on this subject on my website Suite101.com. (Article published by *Parole de Vie* under the number A136). You can reproduce it, as long as you give the references or link to my site.

Question: *How do the Illuminati recognize each other?*

Answer: It is very easy for them, because they have been Illuminati for generations. It is not difficult to recognize family members or close friends. The Illuminati also use tree networks of phone numbers to contact each other when a meeting is scheduled. A month or two before, the governing council schedules a time and place for meetings of the various groups that report to them. They then contact the local leaders (high priests and high priestesses) well in advance, usually a week before. Two days before the meeting, these local leaders notify all the leaders under them. These leaders in turn notify the regular members. The more important a person is in the hierarchy of the group, the more advance notice is given. This is how members recognize their status. People at the bottom of the hierarchy are given very little information because they are less trusted. So they get very little notice of meetings.

Some Illuminati are required to wear special jewelry, such as a ruby ring or an oval emerald, when they have to meet in a public place and have a specific task assigned to them. But most contacts are made through family members or close friends.

When I lived in San Diego, all my family and my four closest friends were members of the Illuminati. So it wasn't hard to contact me. My husband was also a member of the group. The Illuminati have a history of arranged marriages. They don't allow one of their members to marry someone who is not a member of the group. If someone tells you that their spouse is not a member of the group, they can't be a member of the Illuminati themselves. Or they have left the cult. This is an immutable principle. My marriage was arranged by the local ruling council, with another member of the same rank. I didn't want to marry that man because I didn't love him. But I will never forget what Athena, my supervisor at the time (she was the second highest ranking member of the council at the time) said to me: "This is the best choice for you, because he will never be able to control you or harm you. When I was twelve years old, my mother kept telling me, "Never sleep with someone who is lower than you. If you do, they will drag you down. Always choose someone who is higher than you.

My mother was an ambitious woman, to say the least. She was determined to make me succeed in this highly politicized group. I followed her advice. Athena was my girlfriend, and protected me from some of the s--- among the San Diego leaders, especially Jonathan, our leader. She would show me his weaknesses, and teach me how to get around him. She would defend me to him. Otherwise, I couldn't have survived.

These people are definitely not "nice", and they know how to manipulate others in a vicious way. They are only interested in their position, power and money. I voluntarily gave all that up when I left. Sometimes I miss being respected like when I was in a position of responsibility in the group! But I am learning to live in an entirely different way, without having that "family" constantly on my back, controlling me and telling me everything I should do.

Do you know what was the hardest thing for me to experience when I left? My freedom! Not having anyone to tell me what to do anymore. I had to go through a difficult period where I had to learn to adapt. I always felt shaky, and I was always wondering what I should do. It was hard because it was a reflex for me to always talk about my decisions with my management, with Jonathan and with my husband. Believe me if you will, freedom is sometimes hard to live with. It took me a long time to find a balance. I think it's their inability to deal with their freedom that sometimes pushes some of the band members back in, when they're out of it.

I hope this information has been useful to you.

THIRD PART

How the Illuminati run Hollywood

Question: I would think that California is one of the best places for the Illuminati to operate. I'm thinking especially of Hollywood. What do you know about this, about film production, the use of symbols, subliminal messages, and the whole world of show business in general?

Answer: It would take me a few hours to answer you! I'll try to keep it short. The Illuminati believe that you control a country when you control its media. This is one of their clear priorities. Remember that the areas they have decided to invest in to better dominate society are: banking and finance, the media, the judicial and legislative system, the government, and the educational system.

How do they do it? Not by going to a movie producer and saying, "By the way, we're Illuminati, and we'd like you to make a movie to further our agenda. Remember, these are smart people. Instead, they will create a small financial company to fund films that will advance their agenda. They will quietly pick and choose the actors, producers, directors and scripts that interest them, but never publicly say who they really are or what their real goals are.

Money opens all doors, especially in Hollywood. If you have money, you can get almost anything. They know that. They also fund the advertising campaigns for their films. How many Christian films have been able to afford big advertising campaigns in the last twenty years? Very few! Compare that with the advertising campaigns for occult films! No comment!

This has been a long and subtle process, because the Illuminati are patient. They have been working in secret for hundreds of years. They know that the public is slow to accept new ideas, and that it must be done gradually. They call it "sheep driving". That's one of the terms they use for those who are not "enlightened. If you consider the number of occult films that have come out in the last ten years alone, that should be enough to make you think!

Why so many occult films? Why so much awareness of the occult and magic among American youth? Just look at the Saturday morning cartoons on television! I don't allow my kids to watch them, except for the occasional Bugs Bunny! We prefer to rent videos of old classic movies with Audrey Hepburn or John Wayne. I could send you some excellent articles that have thoroughly investigated Walt Disney. He was a member of the Illuminati, and his film Fantasia was designed specifically to program children.

Some movies are designed to promote the Illuminati agenda, like "The Matrix". When I saw this movie, it blew my mind! It refers directly to the Illuminati conditioning process, and it was not fun to watch! Or "Fight Club". I like Brad Pitt and Ed Norton, but this movie clearly shows the military's plan to take over society. Most people don't realize what is happening. Note that the character who embodies the cult of the military symbol is the strongest in the script.

As for the movie "The Labyrinth", I have not seen it, but my husband has. Everything he told me fits exactly with the child programming techniques used by the Illuminati. Any movie that has an occult theme, or features paranormal supernatural phenomena or contact with the spirit world is all designed to further the Illuminati agenda. I don't go to those movies. I have had enough contact with the occult in my past life!

Another example is the sensational presentation of secret rites and other occult rituals on television. Or stories about ghosts and witches. Children's books about witches and witch training are very popular!

The Illuminati strongly believe in Aryan ideology. A movie like "Starship Trooper" has many references to this ideology and many occult symbols. I counted at least 100 of them, and I almost laughed! Someone really got a kick out of pushing the Illuminati agenda when they made this movie!

Many famous actors and actresses are used in films financed by the Illuminati. Some of them know it. Most probably don't know anything, as long as they get their check. Some of them are also Illuminati, although I don't know many of them personally. I won't name the ones I do know. I don't want to risk a libel suit!

Anyway, I was too busy with my job as a trainer, as well as learning about the effects of drugs and other substances on people, to have time to keep up with what was going on in the show business. I'm sorry, but I don't remember many famous names. My life as a trainer and senior programmer was pretty boring. We rarely talked about the media, except that we knew it was one of the ways the Illuminati was setting up their New World Order. That was their real motivation.

I would also like to dispel another misconception that the Illuminati know they are doing evil. When I was a member of the Illuminati, we were completely convinced that our program was very beneficial. As a trainer, I sincerely believed that I was helping others reach their full potential.

I believe that after years of hard work, my intelligence had allowed me to be an excellent leader. I could stand up to Jonathan and other leaders in our group when I thought their decisions were not right, and I stood up for those under me. Others besides me did the same. They honestly think they are doing the right thing. If you told them they were doing wrong, they would be very surprised.

I had to undergo a long therapy and deprogram myself. I got back in touch with reality by hanging out with people who were not in this cult, and by finally understanding that it was all a lie. This was a terrible blow to me! I had dedicated my whole life to helping others get into this glorious New World Order, and I finally discovered that it was all wrong, a horrible exploitation of human beings. I cried and moaned about it for a long time!

Most of the Illuminati I have known were not inherently evil. They were seduced and deceived. Only the top leaders, at the highest level, were probably aware that they were actually doing evil.

PART FOUR

The relationship between Illuminati and Freemasons

Question: Svali, I'm sure most readers would like to know about the relationship between the Illuminati and the Freemasons. What do you know about it? Have the Illuminati infiltrated the Masonic orders?

Answer: The Illuminati and the Freemasons work hand in hand. It doesn't matter if what I say is disturbing, it's a fact. The Masonic Temple in Alexandria, Virginia, is an educational and training center for the Illuminati in the Washington, D.C. area. It was named after the city of Alexandria in Egypt. It is a very important center for Illuminati activities. I myself had to go to the Masonic temple sometimes, for exams, promotion, training, or important ceremonies. The leaders of this Masonic lodge were also Illuminati.

It was the same in every major city I lived in. The leading Freemasons were also high level Illuminati. My maternal grandparents were prominent Masons in the city of Pittsburgh, Pennsylvania (they were [33rd] degree). They were also leaders of the Illuminati in that area.

However, I do not believe that all Freemasons are Illuminati, especially at the lower ranks. At that level, I don't think they know anything about what goes on around midnight in their main temples. Many Masons are also competent businessmen and "good" Christians. But I have never known a Freemason who was not also an Illuminatus, from the [32nd] degree up. It was the Illuminati who created Freemasonry to "cover" their activities.

Question: What exactly does the pyramid on the back of the U.S. dollar bill mean? I'm talking about the pyramid with an eye at the top. Is this a Masonic or Illuminati symbol?

Answer: The pyramid and the "Eye of Horus" on the dollar bill are Illuminati symbols. The pyramid is a geometric figure based on the number 3, a sacred number in ancient religious mysteries. It is the number 3, not 6, that is considered the most sacred number in occultism. The pyramid is also a structure used especially for invoking demons. It is a point of occult activity.

The eye represents the eye of Horus, "the all-seeing eye. The Illuminati place great emphasis on Egyptian magical practices (*the Book of the Dead*, etc.) The eye also represents the fact that no one can escape the scrutiny of magic. The Illuminati consider this eye to be a demonic eye, or the eye of the deity. In Illuminati mythology, this eye can be open or closed, depending on the spiritual time of year, or the spiritual state of the person. Young children are given occult surgery to open their "inner" eye. They are also told that Horus will take away their soul or that this eye will explode if they leave the group or if they speak out. The symbol on the dollar bill serves as a reinforcing message for any Illuminati children who see these bills. It reminds them that someone is watching them.

On the same bill, it is also written in Latin: "Novus Ordo Seclorum", which means "New World Order". This corresponds to the program of the Illuminati. Just think, our ancestors were already thinking about this New World Order in the early 1800s! Didn't I tell you that the Illuminati are patient intellectuals who take the long view? Thomas Jefferson, Benjamin Franklin, Franklin Roosevelt, and others, were top Illuminati. Our country was founded on principles of freedom, but also on the principles of the New World Order.

Question: *How long has this concept of the Illuminati been around? It seems that they have been active for a long time. Did they operate under other names before? What do you know about it?*

Answer: I have been taught that the Illuminati go back to ancient practices that were known from the beginning of historical times, from the time of the Babylonians, who erected ziggurats for their deities, the ones the Illuminati still worship. They are proud of the fact that they have inherited a supposedly unbroken tradition from that time. The names have changed, but the core group has remained the same.

The Illuminati also trace their roots to the mysterious practices of the ancient religions of Egypt, with all their black magic, and the worship of Set, Osiris, Horus and Ra. The Illuminati also believe that they are direct descendants of the Pharaohs of ancient Egypt.

It's hard for me to know how much of this is propaganda, and how much of what they claim is true.

During the Middle Ages, the Knights Templar were also predecessors of the Illuminati, as were the Rosicrucians, and the Celts and their druids. You know, the ones who built Stonehenge in England.

PART FIVE

The relationship between the Illuminati and the CIA, as well as with Russia and China

Svali: I just want your readers to know that I am not an Illuminati expert, nor do I want to be. I am just a survivor, who was part of their group, in a leadership position, but at a local level not very high. I didn't hang out with the rich and famous. But I would hear about what was going on at the highest levels. People gossip a lot in cults too. They are still human beings!

Other people have also come out, and have made revelations. I don't know them personally, but I've heard about them. There's Brice Taylor, who lives in California and North Carolina. There's also Neil Brick from smartnews. I think we can trust him, he's a good person. There's also Caryn stardancer, from Survivorship.org, and Annie mckenna. I think she wrote a book about her experiences, a very good book, published by Paperclip Dolls. There are others, and if you check out Suite101.com, you'll find links to all these resources, and to other survivors. You can also find links to Survivorship.org.

Some of these survivors have posted their own testimonies on the Internet, to help the public know what is going on. So I'm not the only one who has gone out and talked about my experiences. But these are limited to the Washington, D.C. area and the San Diego area, between the years 1957 and 1995. I was in the service of the Illuminati then, completely seduced. Now I deeply regret having participated in all of those things.

Question: How can survivors remain anonymous if they seek help? Couldn't the Illuminati permanently silence programmers or members who have left the group? How far are they willing to go to silence you?

Answer: On my Suite101 website, and in my book, I have written a whole chapter on how to stay safe. Yes, the Illuminati are looking to contact those who have come out. First and foremost through their families.

Remember, we are in the Illuminati from generation to generation. Four years ago, my mother asked me to choose between "return or death. This triggered a deadly program of self-destruction, which they had implanted in me. I think my mother hoped I would come back, but she was wrong. I came very close to death, but God spared me. Then I had to work on dismantling the program. When I left the Illuminati, my boss treated me very arrogantly. He told me that I would be dead within six months, if I remember correctly. He told me that "no one could remember anything, with what I put in them, and still live. This is a direct quote from Jonathan M., my boss, and I hope he reads this article!

But many former members are recaptured or abducted because they continue to call their former friends, or go out alone at night. You wouldn't believe some of the stories I've heard from survivors about going out shopping at two or three in the morning, alone, in deserted places. What on earth are they thinking?

Three years ago, I helped a survivor leave the group. She was literally being persecuted, and was fighting back hard. She ended up holding a gun on the man who was trying to kidnap her. He too had a gun in his hand, and he was threatening her, but she said, "Which one of us do you think is the better shot?" She was a sharpshooter! He gave up. She stayed with me for six months, and now she's free.

Usually, after a while, they give up chasing those who have left, and they get tired of trying to get them back. But I could never live in Washington or San Diego. I would be too likely to run into one of my old acquaintances. It's better to keep some distance. The Illuminati who are where I live now don't know me or care about me. I know a lot of people too. The Illuminati like secrecy. They usually won't do anything in public if you're with people who aren't part of their group. But I've heard of people who have been murdered. That's one of the reasons why I refuse to go on television, or speak in public. I live a very quiet, anonymous life.

Most of the time, when former members are recaptured, it is because they themselves have reconnected with the cult. The temptation to return is sometimes very strong. It must be fought vigorously, especially during the first few years. If you want to know why people who have been abused want to return to their abusers, read an article I wrote called "Trauma Bonds: The Attraction to the Torturer". It is on my website (in English: "Trauma Bonding: The Pull to the Perpetrator").

Question: I want to talk about the Illuminati's political agenda again. What is their relationship with the CIA, FBI, and other secret services? What is the degree of infiltration of these services? What are the real objectives of these secret services?

Answer: They are all infiltrated. I don't think all of them are Illuminati, but a lot of their leaders are. For example, my mother was a friend of Sid Gottlieb, who was in the CIA. The farm I grew up on was only half an hour from his house in Culpeper, Virginia. She also knew the Dulles family (Foster Dulles was U.S. Secretary of State). Many CIA investigators are part of the Illuminati... MK-Ultra (government mind control program)[2] was partly funded by Illuminati money. All these people use the most advanced mind control techniques, believe me, and they start by using them on their own people.

When I lived in San Diego, we were always doing experiments on humans. Jonathan and I were experimenting with the effects of certain drugs that caused trance-like states, combined with programming methods. We would take all the data from our experiments and load it into a database. Yes, the Illuminati are very good at using advanced technology! Then we would ship the data to Langley (the Illuminati's main computer center in Virginia).

Many of the directors and officers of the FBI are also Illuminati. The CIA helped bring German scientists to America after the last world war. Many of them were also high-level leaders among the Illuminati, and they were welcomed with open arms by their American colleagues. They gave their American colleagues all the information they had.

Question: If the political, banking, and military systems in America are largely controlled by the Illuminati, I suppose the same must be true for Eastern Europe, Russia, and the other countries of the former communist bloc. So what about East-West relations? Was Russia, which at the time was the USSR, really the adversary it seemed to be? Was there a Machiavellian plan behind this apparent enmity with Russia?

---

[2] Cf, *MK Ultra, ritual abuse and mind control*, Alexandre Lebreton, Omnia Veritas Ltd, www.omnia-veritas.com.

Answer: Russia has never really been a threat to America. Marxism was founded by the Illuminati, to counterbalance capitalism. The Illuminati believe strongly in the importance of opposing forces, in the necessity of having opposing forces. They see history as a complex game of forces, like a game of chess. So they fund one side, then the other, to take advantage of the chaos and division, and thus move things forward. They go far beyond the game of political parties, and they laugh about it. During all those years (of the Cold War), the big Western financiers met secretly with their Russian or Communist "opponents", and they laughed together about how all those "sheep" could be deceived. I share here what I have been taught, and what I have observed myself.

When the two main Illuminati training groups met in Europe (DELPHI for North America and ORACLE for Europe), all the trainers worked together, whether they were Russian, German, French, English, Canadian or American. This is one of the reasons why the Illuminati is trying to develop language learning as much as possible. I had to learn six languages as a child, and learn to converse with people from all over the world. The Illuminati is a truly international group. National goals must take second place to their supranational goals. The Illuminati also have a habit of traveling a lot to exchange skills. So a Russian trainer might come to the United States for a while to accomplish a specific task, and then return to his country, or vice versa.

Question: China has been making loud booming noises, and it has acquired nuclear weapons, which threaten American cities. Does this all fit with the Illuminati's goals? Are there areas beyond the control of the Illuminati, factors of uncertainty?

Answer: It's been five years since I left the Illuminati. So my information is getting a little old. But the development of Chinese military power is part of their plan. There are members of their group who are Asian, and they are very opportunistic. The eastern mafias are very much linked to Illuminati activities. The only uncertain factors for the Illuminati are how ordinary citizens will react. They cannot predict this. However, the Illuminati leadership devises several scenarios, and tries to anticipate the appropriate response, should the citizens behave unexpectedly.

I was told that the Illuminati planned to make their entire program public by the year 2020. I don't know if this information is reliable, or if it's just propaganda. It is also possible that they have changed the date since I was a member of this group.

Question: *Svali, you've spoken to us before about mind control techniques, and about survivors who have published their testimony. One of these recent testimonies is that of Cathy O'Brian*

(www.vegan.swinternet.co.uk/articles/conspiracies/cathyansmark.html and www.trance-formation.com).

She seems to be one of the victims of the CIA's mind control programs. Her story is very similar to yours, in terms of technology and techniques. Do you think there might be a connection with the Illuminati?

Answer: I've said it before, the CIA and the Illuminati work together. It is clear. The leaders of the CIA are also high-level Illuminati. I told you about Foster Dulles and Sid Gottlieb, whom I knew personally as a child and young adult. The scientists who developed the MK-Ultra program and other government mind control programs were Illuminati who came from Nazi Germany. This is why you will find that the victims of mind control always speak German, or have a disassociated part of their personality that speaks with a German accent. They imitate their torturers, which is very common.

You can tell that the CIA and the Illuminati are working hand in hand. I know that various Illuminati groups throughout the United States send the data they collect from their experiments to the central computer center in Langley, Virginia. Yes, experiments are still being conducted on human beings, especially in the area of mind control! They did not stop with the end of the Second World War!

SIXTH PART

Why is there so little media coverage of ritual abuse and mind control?

Question: *I find it very surprising that these issues of ritual abuse and mind control are hardly discussed in the press, given the large amount of evidence available.*

Answer: My answer is going to sound really cynical. But I am not surprised by this. Because the Illuminati boast that their best protection is the ignorance and disbelief of the public. They also know how to run their own press campaigns, which are very effective. For example, I knew a reporter for the San Diego Union Tribune (his name initials are M.S.) who wrote articles about ritual abuse and mind control. He was part of the Illuminati. His articles were a typical model of how the Illuminati operate.

He was interviewing doctors who were supposedly respected specialists in the field. These men had degrees. They would give the rational and considered opinion of an expert, and come to the conclusion that no reasonable and logical human being can believe in the existence of ritual abuse. Furthermore, they believe that the doctors and therapists who treat the so-called victims of ritual abuse are nothing more than charlatans who take advantage of the poor, naive people who are exploited by these particularly vicious and self-interested people.

He then denounced those who claimed that ritual abuse really existed, making them look like narrow-minded mental patients. He also denounced the "fraudulent" and "exploitative" behavior of the doctors and therapists who treated them. He portrayed them as practically greedy, greedy for gain, and plunged into all sorts of mental delusions. He portrayed all those poor families torn apart by those awful therapists who were accused of injecting those ideas of ritual abuse into the heads of those poor victims.

All of this was wrapped up in the seemingly rational, logical, and compassionate comments of a member of the federal social services, who said how tragic it all was, concluding that something absolutely had to be done.

M.S. never mentions that the doctors who treat survivors of ritual abuse get paid very little, and even work for free, to help these people break the chains of a lifetime. M.S. never interviews the 85% of psychological workers who know that ritual abuse exists or who believe in its existence. He only interviews the small minority who agree with his ideas.

So we know that the media is often very biased!

Question: But since there is so much evidence, why aren't more people interested in the Illuminati?

Answer: Simply because people can't and won't believe that the Illuminati exist, and that everything I'm telling you is really happening. I am a committed Christian. In the book of Revelation, it says that just before Jesus returns, people will live as if nothing is going to happen, and say that everything is normal, despite the clear evidence to the contrary. Even if you showed someone a video taken during ritual abuse, they would say, "It must be a fake. People don't do things like that. You could show someone a place with buried bones, pentagrams and other satanic symbols, they would say, "Oh, it's just kids having fun!" You could still show them pictures of the tunnels built near Los Alamos, they would say, "That's irrelevant. It must be about some government project!" Show them the scars that the survivors have on their bodies, cigarette burn marks from when they were children, or whip marks on their backs, they would say, "Are you sure they didn't do that to themselves?"

The evidence is there. But, in my opinion, people, in general, don't want to know. Even when you put the evidence in front of them, they look away.

The Franklin case is an example. Yet there was no lack of evidence! Or all the documents about the MK-Ultra project that have been made public, and which have been proven to be true. People ignore them. I believe that the media that refuses to admit to ritual abuse is taking advantage of the fact that many people, deep down, do not want to know the reality. In fact, how can they admit that human nature is so inherently evil, unless they really believe in God, or have irrefutable proof? Men still want to believe that their species is always capable of the best, not the worst!

Question: *You have probably heard of the "Bohemian Grove". What do you know about it? Is there a connection with the Illuminati?*

Answer: I have never heard of the "Bohemian Grove". Remember that my position did not allow me to know everything! Most of my contacts were in Germany. I was never prostituted. Rather, it was me teaching others to do so. I have never been to Bohemia, and I don't know anything about this "Grove". I'm sorry I can't answer you.

But if you asked me about the Masonic temple in Alexandria, Virginia, or the "Institute" in Charlottesville, or the little grove I know in Canada with a bronze statue of Baal, I could answer you. I'm sorry I don't have anything to tell you on this topic. But if the "Bohemian Grove" has anything to do with the occult, the Illuminati certainly know about it!

PART SEVEN

Symbols and marks of the Illuminati
Degree of infiltration of the society

Question: Yes, tell us more about all this: your contacts in Germany, the Masonic temple, "The Institute," and the statue of Baal in Canada! Also tell us what the main symbols and marks of the Illuminati are, apart from the pyramid and the eye of Horus. Can the Illuminati sometimes act recklessly?

Answer: To answer you completely, I would have to make you read my complete biography! I have sometimes had the idea of writing it, but I don't think many would read it. I'm serious, it's not about false modesty. Besides, I don't think people want anything to do with the Illuminati, even if they learn something about it. Forgive my cynicism, but this is my life experience!

The Illuminati don't care about the testimonies that are written and those who denounce them, because they count on the fact that most people don't believe those who write them. They know how to do press campaigns! Have you read the recent articles in *Newsweek* and *Time*, which consider the existence of the Illuminati as a ridiculous imaginary conspiracy? Do you know who owns the capital of these magazines?

Five years ago, at a board meeting, I heard the Illuminati scoff at all the revelations that were coming to light. I don't think they've changed their minds now. If people started to believe all this, and if they started to act, I would be very surprised, and very happy.

I'll give you an example. Two years ago, I was trying to find a publisher for my book about how the Illuminati programs people. I wanted the book to help doctors who treat survivors. But I couldn't find anyone willing to publish it! I was told that it was too controversial a subject, and that there was "not a big enough market for this kind of book. It's sad, but that's what happened!

Yet, I believe that God is completely directing the history of the world. I have denounced the Illuminati, and I have published my book on the

Internet for free. I want those who deal with the survivors to realize what they have been through. It's hard to help those who have come out of this if you don't understand the physical and emotional trauma they had to go through.

I'll now return to your questions.

The National Council of the Illuminati in Germany is called the "Bruderheist". It meets in the Black Forest. This region is considered by them to be the center of the world, and an intense center of psychic and spiritual energies. I have met some of the most depraved and evil people I have ever known there! They support the Nazis. But, compared to them, the Nazis look like good people! They're still out there, still manipulating people, still running the banks, still funneling their dirty money to Brussels, Switzerland, Cairo, Egypt.

Canada also has a very large group of Illuminati and Templars. These are two groups that work hand in hand. They worship ancient deities. The bronze (or gold?) statue of Baal is in the middle of a sacred grove on a large private property between Quebec City and Montreal. I was 12 years old when I went there. So I don't remember all the details well. But the ceremonies held there attracted a large crowd, people dressed all in white. There were lots of flowers and fruit, votive offerings, singing, and then the final sacrifice in the arms of the statue.

Regarding the symbols and marks of the Illuminati, let me first remind you that they are the most careful people on earth! They try never to leave a trace! But you can see most of their symbols on television or in movies. They are also very attached to the idea of a military government. These people are extremely militaristic.

One of their main symbols is the phoenix (the mythical bird that dies by fire and rises from the ashes). It is one of their main military and spiritual symbols. The German eagle is also an important sign. Some companies use the phoenix in their logo, red on a black background, or the opposite. This is a very important sign, because the Illuminati use many rituals that evoke resurrection. During these rituals, people are taken to a state very close to death. Then they are "resurrected" and told that Baal, or some other god, has "given them life" and that they owe it to him (and to the group) to be alive. The phoenix is thus a very important sign.

They also use butterflies and the rainbow a lot. Why butterflies? Because the Illuminati have invented, together with the CIA, a method of mental programming called "Monarch", like the name of these big butterflies. They also use as symbols some special jewelry. Video games (like Ultima, for example) are full of Illuminati symbols, like magic gems. I don't play these video games...

The tiara, or crown bearing 13 precious stones, with a diamond in the center, is the symbol of the coming reign of the "chosen one.

Another symbol of the Illuminati is the Star of David. Believe me, it is one of their most powerful religious symbols. They represent it inside a circle. They call it the "Great Seal of Solomon. It is used in the most important ceremonies, to summon demons.

We must also mention earth, water, and fire. These three elements are used in many ceremonies. Check it out, and you will see that many cartoons often use these symbols. You'd be surprised to find out! The movie "The Fifth Element" was based on this concept.

The Illuminati use a lot of signs and symbols that appeal to Greek and Roman mythologies. Their mental programming methods also draw heavily on these mythologies. Most "programmed" people have an internal structure with a Greek or Roman temple.

They also use the lightning symbol. Many modern logos depict a lightning bolt. I saw a recent copy of *Time* magazine, whose ads were filled with Illuminati symbols. Another important symbol is a head with a computer in it. It represents "delta programming".

Question: *Tell us yourself about things we haven't talked about yet in these interviews, maybe things that I missed, about the New World Order, for example...*

Answer: The Illuminati are pedophiles. They torture and abuse little children. They teach them from an early age to become criminals themselves. This alone should be absolutely stopped!

They control the pornographic industry, with the Maffia. They make a lot of money in drug and arms trafficking, and in human trafficking, i.e. in slavery! Yes, we continue today, at the beginning of the [21st century,] to buy and sell human beings!

They run everything that makes money and everything that is evil! If there is any profit to be made on the backs of human suffering, you can find the Illuminati in it!

Since they have a lot of money, they can afford lawyers who can convict anyone who tries to expose them.

They have infiltrated our government, and every government in the world. They have also infiltrated the judicial system and the legislative system. They have infiltrated the media. They run all our financial institutions.

They have no scruples and are very ambitious. They will not hesitate to suppress all those who oppose them. They are the ones who invented mental programming, with the CIA.

Do you want to know more? Let me just tell you a little more about what they look like!

They are working to prepare for the coming of a new world leader, who will bring the world into a new reign of joy, prosperity, and rewards for their followers. Almost a type of heaven on earth! Of course, it will still be a reign of brutality. Those who would oppose this reign will be hunted down. They will have to convert or be put to death. But their followers will be so happy and content with this new regime that they will be convinced that everyone will come and join them. It sounds incredible, but it is true!

In this New World Order, people will be given new jobs, and positions of responsibility. The Illuminati believe that their children are the best, the brightest and the most educated. They will form the intellectual elite who will lead the masses of those who are less intelligent and less "gifted.

This is what the Illuminati really believe. They worship Plato's ideal Republic, which is the model for their New World Order.

But there is also the other side of the coin!

They are very arrogant, which could be their downfall. They consider most people as "sheep" without intelligence. They are full of pride and believe they are invulnerable. They consider anything the press says about them a mere mosquito bite. But arrogant people make mistakes. They are less and less reluctant to reveal themselves these days.

They believe that they can defeat God, which is a huge mistake on their part! God can change the course of history. He has already done so, in the hope that some of these people will come out of it. God is merciful.

Most of the Illuminati are themselves wounded and seduced victims. They themselves have suffered many abuses. They do not know that it is possible to leave this group. There is a lot of discontent in the ranks of the Illuminati. If they knew that it is possible to escape, without being put to death, we would see a mass exodus. Many of the trainers I knew were not at all happy with what they were doing, while being vicious pedophiles. I could tell by the signs, when they sighed silently, or by the looks, that they did not approve of what they were being asked to do. They did their work with resignation, hoping for a promotion. You know what one of the biggest carrots offered to those who want promotions is in this group. It's the knowledge that they'll be able to avoid torturing people, or being tortured themselves. And it's true! You can only be tortured by someone whose position is higher than yours. So everybody wants to move up. The higher you go, the less people there are above you! It is true that there are people who torture others by choice, and that motivates them to seek promotion. But that's not the case for everyone!

As more and more people leave the Illuminati, more and more doctors, therapists and church leaders are becoming aware of the sophisticated mind control methods that were used to control these people. So they are learning how to deprogram these survivors.

But it is prayer that can bring about the greatest victories. My greatest hope is that everyone I have known in this group, including all the leaders and all the people who have hurt me so much at times, can one day leave. If they could know that it was possible, I truly believe they would leave!

Question: I have sometimes seen Clinton, and even Prince William of England, make a certain hand sign (index and little fingers extended, other fingers closed). Does this gesture have a hidden meaning?

Answer: This is an old sign of greeting and recognition between Satanists. But the Illuminati are usually more subtle than that, and do not make this gesture in public.

PART EIGHT

The Fourth Reich

Question: When you describe the Illuminati, it sounds a lot like what was going on in Germany during the Third Reich. I clearly recognize in them the behavior and goals of the Nazis. It seems that Germany is regaining a dominant role in European unification. We are seeing the formation of a European army, a European Rapid Intervention Force, and an International Tribunal. How far will this finally go?

Answer: The Illuminati have a term for the New World Order. They refer to it as the "Fourth Reich". I am serious. Many Illuminati are mentally programmed for this Fourth Reich. Yes, Germany and Europe will dominate the world economy. The U.S. economy will regress for a while, then recover with the help of Europe.

Question: Revelation paints a pretty bleak picture of how this is all going to end. But does that have any effect on the Illuminati agenda? They certainly know the prophecies in the Bible, which speak of their final defeat. Are they trying to use these prophecies to their advantage, by deceiving human beings?

Answer: In fact, they deny the prophecies. They believe that history can be changed, and that the revelations of the apostle John are only one possible interpretation of the future. They know about Revelation, but they do not attach much importance to it.

Remember that some of the leading Illuminati are already in power. They control the world's finances and have immense wealth. Some of them own several large estates around the world, and they have everything they desire, not to mention the pleasure of controlling millions of human beings. They believe in their intellectual power, and are convinced that they will form the elite of the New World Order. They will be the "good people" of tomorrow. But they are Luciferians. It is therefore normal for them to believe that the Bible says things that are not true.

If you were to talk to them openly about these things, they would laugh in your face and say, "But the New Order is already in place! It's just not fully manifested!"

The Illuminati have been in power in the world for several hundred years. They will tell you that no God has struck them down yet. They may even believe that they are doing God's will on earth. Remember, they believe they are serving "God," as Christians might believe!

They would say to you: "Why would God have given man such latent abilities, if He had not wanted him to discover them and use them fully? Is it not criminal to neglect and not to develop all these capacities? Is it not criminal not to help the human race to progress and become better?" this is what they would tell you, trying to persuade you.

They believe that they are basically good, and that they are doing a good job, even if the means used are sometimes very hard to bear. They "pull the weeds" by getting rid of the weak and unfit. They want to produce a superior human race. I know that what I am saying sounds like cat food, but the Illuminati are sincerely convinced that they are right. For them to see themselves under the judgments of Revelation, they would have to begin to understand that they are doing evil and that they are evil, which they are not.

I hope what I'm saying helps you understand better. I think the Illuminati see themselves riding white horses and not black horses. Do you understand the power of seduction? But I am now a Christian, and I have completely rejected everything I previously believed in this cult.

PART NINE

Ritual sacrifices
Relationships with demons
Changes in physical form

Questions: Svali, you have already spoken to us about ritual sacrifice. You talked about animal sacrifices. Can you give us more details on these subjects?

Answer: I hate to go into sensationalism with awful details, but I'll talk about it a bit.

First, remember that the Illuminati are concerned with six main areas. Sacrifices are practiced within the "spiritual realm. But the spiritual realm is only one of their areas of focus. My domain was the Science domain. I laughed at those of us who specialized in the spiritual realm. Yet we all had to go through certain "spiritual" rituals on special holidays. But I tried to go as little as possible. They were always horrible, crude, brutal things. But they were considered important.

In the Celtic branch of this spiritual realm, it is believed that power is passed on as one passes from life to death. The Illuminati therefore have certain rituals in which a child, or an adult, is tied up and an animal is bled to death by being placed on its body. They believe that the person who is tied up receives power when the spirit of the dead animal "enters" them. It is traumatic enough to have an animal bleeding to death on your body! Imagine the impression made on a young child, especially if they are threatened that they will be bled to death if they speak!

I must also tell you about opening "portals" to enter "another dimension. I know this sounds like science fiction, but the Illuminati actually believe that there are other spiritual dimensions and that in order to enter one of them, you have to make a major ritual sacrifice just to "open the portal. Usually several animals have to be sacrificed. I have also witnessed animal sacrifices made to be protected from demons. A circle is then drawn with blood, so that the demons cannot enter the circle.

The Illuminati absolutely believe in the existence of a spiritual world. For hundreds of years, they have codified their rituals, based on ancient occult rituals. They believe they can control these powers. I believe they are seduced (they are the ones being controlled).

They also make sacrifices during certain annual festivals. I witnessed the killing of an animal, directly by the power of thought. I cannot explain what I saw. I have also witnessed human sacrifices, but these are very rare. I think I have seen two or three human sacrifices in all. The others were staged.

The Illuminati do not want to sacrifice their children in general. They want their new generation to grow up and continue their practices. I have also heard that they buy children in other countries to sacrifice them, or that they kidnap homeless people for this purpose, but I have never seen this myself.

Most often, animals are sacrificed during their rituals. This is what I have seen. Because of my duties as a senior trainer, I have had to witness, but very rarely, human sacrifices. They are rare, but horrific. The trainers did not usually push people to death, they watched for certain signs of stress. Their doctors also knew how to use certain new drugs to create states of dazedness, and to control or suppress the most obvious signs of stress (increased heart rate and breathing, tremors, pupil dilation).

Some inexperienced trainers might not be able to observe these signs and let someone go completely downhill. It's a terrible thing to "work" with someone and have them lose their mind for good! These people then become vegetables, or scream for hours on end.

Sometimes we had to "get rid" of these "failures" in training by injecting them with air or insulin. We would then make up the death as a "fatal accident" or let their bodies burn in an induced fire. May God forgive me for the few occasions when I was directly involved in such things and was forced to act. Today, I deeply regret it. Some people could be kind and sympathetic. Moreover, the trainer himself knew that this could happen to him too. So he tried to do his job well.

All failures were severely punished. One of my tasks as a trainer was to train the young trainers to use the various drugs to mask the effects of stress, and to recognize the subtle signs of distress. (Sigh!) Are these failures also considered "sacrifices"? I believe so, even though they were not rituals as such, because everything was done in laboratories, in white coats and with medical equipment.

Question: *Svali, I would like to ask you another question. There are stories circulating that the Illuminati are controlled by aliens, specifically by a reptilian race from another dimension. What do you think about this?*

Answer: My answer will undoubtedly make some people angry, but I don't want to offend anyone! I have never seen aliens. But I have witnessed some mental programming to make people believe that they have seen aliens. The Illuminati wanted to cover up their mental programming experiments if the victims remembered anything. None of the high officials I knew believed in the existence of aliens. But I never asked them.

I personally believe that this reptilian race thing is really just a manifestation of demons. I have also witnessed changes in physical form, under the influence of demons, and other similar things. Some people may accuse me of believing in the existence of demons, and that this is as absurd as believing in extraterrestrials.

So I would like to point out what the Illuminati really believe. They know that there are spiritual or supernatural beings. But they believe they can control them. I know that some readers will tell me that the changes in physical form were just hallucinations caused by the drugs that were taken during a ritual. I leave it up to each person to decide what they want to believe, depending on the limits of their personal comfort. But I can assure you that no aliens visited Washington or San Diego when I was there. At least, I have never personally seen one.

PART TEN

Further details on the changes in physical form caused by demons

Question: Tell me more about these physical changes. I've heard about this before. Doesn't this only happen during rituals? I have heard that some politicians can move in space. When you say that these changes are caused by demons, are you talking about specific demons? Could it be that these "demons" are in fact some of the aliens who influence the Illuminati?

Answer: Since you're talking about fitness changes, I'll give you some more information. But I will also tell you what I personally believe. I can't help but talk about some fundamental aspects of my Christian faith when it comes to demons.

I was raised in a group that glorifies all things demonic. Then, a few years ago, I became a Christian. I honestly believe that without my faith in Jesus Christ, I would never have been able to get out of the Illuminati. One of the reasons I don't fear for my life when I testify is because I believe that God is able to protect me.

His love is the opposite of the cruelty and wickedness I have seen in this group. His infinite compassion, tenderness and purity are the opposite of the darkness and sexual abuse that accompanies the Illuminati's ritualistic ceremonies. I believe that God has forgiven my past. I have sincerely asked Him for forgiveness. Without it, I would never have been able to go on living, remembering all the things I did to others, such as drugging young girls to become prostitutes for the cult, just to name one example.

I gave up my whole past life. Only with Christ could I receive the love, forgiveness and healing I needed. My soul was disgusted to the core to have lived in the depths of life and to have seen the cruelty that human beings are capable of towards their fellow man.

I certainly believe that demons exist in the occult world. They do exist. They are organized in a spiritual hierarchy, a hierarchy that the

Illuminati are trying to imitate on the physical plane.

There are principalities, and lower demons. They control the gateways to other spiritual dimensions, which should be of no interest to human beings at all. These things are extremely destructive.

The changes in physical form usually took place during an occult ceremony. Those who changed their form in this way had completely given themselves over to the activity of demons. These men changed into animals for a certain period of time, or into other hideous creatures, which were definitely not aliens! It was the activity of the demons that allowed human beings to reveal the demonic realm in this way, also distorting what they saw.

I have also seen people become temporarily "blind" because of the influence of demons. I have seen animals killed by a spiritual power, when several people made a circle and concentrated their energy to kill the animal. These people were not aliens. I was raised with some of them. My own mother did this. She was not an alien, though. I myself have sometimes participated in such things. I am not an alien, but a wounded human being.

I also believe that demons can have sex with humans, because the Book of Genesis talks about it. God totally forbids this.

In fact, the divine covenants presented in the Bible are the opposite of the dark covenants practiced by the Illuminati. I found an abundant source of healing when I saw in the Scriptures how God views our world and how He deals with the spiritual world. He will have the last word. He is winning the battle.

I will tell you about a dream I had two years ago. I was standing in a large, circular room with rows of seats. On the wall was a large representation of the world, with a garland. The room was filled with people in long robes. I knew I was standing in front of the Supreme World Council, the one who will rule the world when the New World Order is installed. They were pointing at me, telling me that I had betrayed their cause, and that I should die.

The darkness and oppression in that room was intolerable. I was suffocating in this atmosphere. One of the leaders came forward, and told me that I must die the death of traitors, unless I returned to the "family". I fought the evil temptation to give in, to save my life. Inwardly, I cried out to the Lord and said, "Jesus, save me! Immediately, the love and peace of the Lord invaded my heart. I was no longer afraid. I said, "No, because you are defeated, even if you don't know it. You can kill my body, but I serve a God who has defeated you, and who has defeated everyone in this room.

I woke up at that moment, filled with joy. You can see why I am not afraid to answer your questions about my past. I believe in a God who is greater than all the plans of these evil men. They can plot as much as they want. But all their plans will eventually be destroyed.

So ask me anything you want, and I'll tell you everything I remember. I don't mind revealing what these people do. I know, however, that I am under no illusions as to what the general public will make of my revelations.

I respect your desire to investigate, and your openness to all my answers. But what I can tell you, and all my past experience has confirmed it, is that I have seen demons at work, not aliens or a reptilian race from outer space! Even if aliens did exist, I wonder if they could be as evil and cruel as the demons I have seen at work, especially against Bible-bound Christians.

PART ELEVEN

Evidence of the Illuminati and their weaknesses

Question: *Svali, have you ever publicly told your story, or is this the first time you have done so?*

Answer: I have never talked much about all the demonic aspects, because it is a controversial subject. I've talked to my husband, my doctor, and a close friend about my experiences. I am not really a "public figure". I just posted a few articles on Suite101.com, to help those who wanted to get out of this cult.

I hate sensationalism because it takes us away from the real issues, especially the issue of children being tortured and abused and the need to stop all that abuse. Whether you talk about demons or aliens, the point is that there are people filled with evil who are using little children and profiting from their suffering. That's why I testified against the Illuminati.

Question: *I am sure that many readers will tell you that this is just science fiction, and wonder if it is all true. They would like you to give them specific evidence. What would you tell them?*

Answer: I'll tell them, "Arrange to attend one of their ceremonies, and you'll have plenty of evidence!" Except that I really don't wish anyone to attend these horrors! Besides, beings that are spirits leave no physical traces. But I think it's interesting that throughout history, there are people who have written accounts of these same phenomena. Could it be that everything they wrote was wrong? Could these people all be pathological liars, throughout the centuries? If you go to Africa, you will hear about sorcerers who change their physical form and transform themselves into animals. In Africa, they don't talk about "dissociation of the personality"! You can ask people, and they were fully aware when they witnessed these things!

This is also happening in South America and Asia. How can these things happen in the same way, all over the world, in groups that have no contact with each other?

Do demons leave a trace, a mark, or physical evidence? I say clearly, "No!" But they do leave an indelible impression on all who have witnessed their action and manifestation. There are written records of these things, as far back as the medieval period. I never took pictures when it happened. So people have to make do with oral testimonies. Whether they believe them or not, it doesn't really matter to me. I know what I saw.

Question: *To conclude this first series of interviews, could you tell us about the weaknesses of the Illuminati? What are the areas where they are vulnerable? Is there any way to stop them? Will humanity ever be able to say, "It's over!"*

Answer: Their main weakness is their arrogance. I think I mentioned this before. These people think they are untouchable. This can cause them to be careless.

The only way to stop them, eventually, would be for Christians to take this problem really seriously, and start organizing to prevent the Illuminati from taking over completely. But that would take a miracle. It would take prayer and God's guidance. Maybe then we can stop them. I hope so with all my heart.

It would also be necessary to stop pornography, child prostitution, and the drug and arms trades, because these are the areas where the Illuminati make the most money. Maybe that would slow them down, because it would deprive them of a huge source of profit. But I honestly believe that it would be as difficult to stop all of this as it would be to stop the Illuminati themselves.

To be honest, I don't know what could really stop them. I have testified against them to try to stop them. I have been to the police on several occasions, I even gave my video testimony during a trial. (I was questioned by five lawyers, and it lasted three hours). I knew that my former boss would receive a copy of this video. I was even tempted for a moment to smile and wave at him and say, "Hi, Jonathan! But I thought I might have gone a little too far.

I have encouraged other Illuminati to come out, and I have helped a few survivors get out, and find a safe haven somewhere. I believe we all need to do something to fight the Illuminati, by letting the Lord lead us. As I write easily, this is one of the ways I have chosen to fight.

Question: *Do you have any comments on topics I haven't mentioned, or that you would like to address yourself? Please feel free to do so.*

Answer: If you could hear the sobs of a child being tortured, brutalized or raped by adults, or the screams of terror of a child being psychologically abused, you would do anything to stop the abuse! They use children as young as three or four years old to make pornographic films. These children are beaten to a pulp if they refuse. Little ones who are just starting to walk are forced to witness brutality. They are then given a whip and told to hit the victims themselves, or they will be whipped themselves. Often the children hesitate, refuse to do so, and the adults present hit these children until they obey. Big tears run down their cheeks, and they reluctantly do what the adults command. It is unbearably cruel!

They put electric collars around the necks of small children, and send them an electric shock if they try to escape. They are treated like animals. The adults and other children who witness this laugh at them and laugh out loud. These poor children will vomit in a corner out of fear and self-loathing.

These are memories that all survivors who have left the Illuminati hold in their hearts. That is why I write and testify against these people, to expose them. I pray with all my heart that they can be stopped. I wish I could get rid of these memories, but they are there. I wish I didn't have these images in my memory, but they don't go away.

Question: *Svali, would you be willing to answer readers' questions, which could lead to other possible articles? I think they would have questions for you, probably about some of the details of your testimony.*

Answer: I would prefer that they send you their questions, and that you forward them to me. I don't want to receive insulting or threatening letters! Because the topics I address are controversial. They are things that are considered "politically incorrect" and should not be discussed in general.

I'm sure some people will criticize me for trying to capture attention. It's true that when I speak to students, or when I give lectures, the listeners are captivated, and, moreover, it's more pleasant for me! I already attract attention to myself by the various articles I publish (on other topics than those we have discussed!) In addition, I earn money with these articles, which is not the case when I testify against the Illuminati...

So you can be sure that I am not trying to draw attention to myself. What I want is to denounce these people. Some readers will believe me, others will not. I accept this without any problem. If some people want to give vent to their disbelief, that is their business. But I personally do not want to receive insults and curses. Because I sometimes receive letters like that, written by people with bad manners!

I have two university degrees. I had to get them because I was part of this cult. They don't let ignorant people run them. So I won't retract anything I said to you! You can send me as many emails as you want with questions from readers, and I will be more than happy to tell you what all these b....ds are capable of, and what they are. I know I'm using an un-Christian term here, but God appreciates honesty, doesn't he? I am just describing them as they really are. I know I still have some growing to do in terms of forgiveness, as you can see!

Question: *Svali, thank you for taking the time to share your experiences with us. I am sure it has not been easy or pleasant for you. I wish you and your family the best. Perhaps many people will read these articles and pass them on to others. Maybe we will be able to stop the atrocities and the abuse of children. Maybe we will be able to put an end to the Illuminati one day. It is never too late. Thank you very much for these interviews, Svali.*

TWELFTH PART

The top of the pyramid

Question: Svali, I'm sure all of our readers are asking a very important question: Who is leading the Illuminati? Who are the people at the top of the pyramid?

Answer: I don't know where to begin to answer you! It depends on the level at which one places oneself. I would like to draw from my memories to make a small map of the Illuminati. But they are not very pleasant memories! I'll try to give you some names too, but I want to be very careful. If I give too many names, I might trigger severe attacks from the members of this group!

To describe the structure of the Illuminati and how they are hierarchical, I will start with the base of the pyramid.

The first level is the city level. There are Illuminati in every city. In most metropolitan areas, they form ten to thirteen "brother" groups. It depends on the size of the city. The larger the city, the more sister groups there are. There are Illuminati groups in every major American city, as well as in every major European city. This first level is called the "low level" or the "anarchic level" (etymologically speaking, the lowest level). Each group is under the authority of a high priest or high priestess. It also includes two or three formators. The others are charged with various functions. The different brother groups meet on rare occasions. They know each other, but each group is relatively independent. All groups report to a metropolitan leadership council.

The second level is the metropolitan leadership council. It has authority over all the local groups in its constituency, as well as over small groups scattered in rural areas.

A metropolitan board of directors consists of 13 members: a "Baal" (chief), two assistants to the chief, four administrators who handle finances and day-to-day business, and six senior trainers, who direct and train all trainers in the metropolitan area. The "Baalim" and their assistants report to a regional governing council.

At the third level are the regional governing boards. The United States has been divided into seven distinct regions. Each region is headed by a thirteen-member council, which oversees all the metropolitan councils within its jurisdiction. The Illuminati organization is very similar to that of Amway, or of well-organized businesses. Each member is given the details of the specific tasks assigned to them. In general, these regional councils consist of thirteen seats, or chairs, according to the various areas of interest to the Illuminati: military (2 chairs), spiritual (2 chairs), knowledge (2 chairs), finance (2 chairs), training and education (2 chairs), and science (2 chairs). With the chairman of the council, this makes 13 members.

These regional councils represent the different areas of interest that the Illuminati deal with. Chair holders change as promotions or demotions occur.

The presidents of all the regional councils report to a National Council. All European nations also have a National Council, as do Mexico, Canada, Russia and China.

The National Council deals with the same areas of interest, but with one important difference: they are usually composed of members of old financial dynasties, such as the Rockefeller, Mellon, Carnegie, Rothschild, etc. families. I know I shouldn't name them, but I do. In France and England, the Rothschild family has a permanent seat on the National Councils of those countries, as do descendants of royal families, or members of reigning royal families. A descendant of the Habsburg dynasty also has a permanent seat in his country. In the United States, the Rockefeller family has a permanent seat on the National Council.

All the National Councils depend on the Supreme World Council. This Council is the prototype of the one that will dominate the world when the New World Order is fully established. It meets regularly to discuss financial issues, policies, and to resolve any difficulties. Again, you will find members of the old financial dynasties.

Now you can see why the Illuminati have been virtually untouchable for centuries! The leading members, at the highest level, are extremely wealthy and powerful. I hope that what I am revealing to you will give you a better understanding of this system.

Where did I get this information? I was a member of a metropolitan board of directors, as a lead trainer. So I was meeting with members of the regional board that I reported to. In addition, all the children of the

Illuminati are taught who their senior leaders are. They are also asked to swear loyalty to them and the New World Order.

Question: What is the degree of involvement of the European royal families in the Illuminati? What is their real power, and what is their relationship with the United States, especially in the political and financial fields? Are we still ruled by kings?

Answer: It is not easy to answer, but I will try. The leaders of the Illuminati claim to be descended from royal families themselves, as well as families that have been continuously involved in the occult for generations.

So there are two definitions of what we mean by "royal families". First, there are the royal families that everyone knows. But there are also the secret royal families, those with blue blood, who possess great occult power. Sometimes, the two lines merge, as in the case of the Prince of Wales.

I don't know which of these two lines really holds the power. I was just a little slave doing her job seriously. But here's what I understood: In Germany, it is the members of the Hanover and Habsburg families who rule the "Bruderheist" (German National Council). They are also considered to have the strongest occult power for generations. The British royal family is just below them in the hierarchy. Occultly, in Britain, the Rothschilds are superior to the Royal Family. They rule Britain, along with the Royal Family, even though Parliament officially rules!

In France, it is the descendants of the royal family who hold the power on the occult plane. But again, the Rothschild family is more powerful than any of them. The American Illuminati are considered "younger" and less powerful than their European colleagues. For this reason, the children of the American Illuminati are always sent to Europe for part of their training. European training is considered better. In addition, American Illuminati families want to renew their affiliation with their European elders.

All the Illuminati in Europe are led by the Illuminati of Germany, France and Great Britain. These three countries form a triumvirate that rules Europe. Russia is considered important because it has the greatest military power and houses the most important Illuminati military groups. The Illuminati have promised Russia the fourth place in the New World Order, even before the United States. Because Russia, and the former USSR, have been more cooperative than the United States in carrying out the Illuminati agenda, over the past decades.

In the world leadership of the Illuminati, therefore, you find members of ancient ruling families, as well as members of newer families. Marxism does not exist for the Illuminati. In the order of global preeminence, you'll find Russia, then China, then the United States. But many of the American Illuminati leaders will emigrate to Europe when the New World Order is established. Many already have property there. They will change their nationality overnight.

I have told you the little that I remember. I would have liked to have studied all this more when I was in the cult, but at that time I was too busy keeping myself alive!

THIRTEENTH PART

The United Nations, or the Supreme World Council

Question: Svali, what role will the United Nations play in the future, and how do you see that role? What is the Illuminati timetable?

Answer: The United Nations was created to overcome one of the biggest obstacles to the implementation of the New World Order. For this to happen, there must be a military order, and the Illuminati must impose their dictatorship. This obstacle is nationalism and patriotism. This is why the New World Order concept was not popular when it was first introduced. It took years for the media to brainwash and destroy the sense of national pride through subtle media campaigns.

The Illuminati agenda is to set up an organization that will foreshadow what will happen when the Supreme World Council officially takes over. Every ambassador to the United Nations has done something to curry favor with the Illuminati and receive a reward from them. Or they are high profile individuals who have been appointed to make the organization look good. The Illuminati and world leaders decided to create a United Nations and worked hard to impose it on the world. Franklin Roosevelt was their man in the United States, as he did much to get the United Nations accepted by Americans. He, and his wife Eleanor were very committed Illuminati. So was Shirley Temple Black. In fact, most of our Presidents, since the beginning of the last century, have been Illuminati, or sworn to support their agenda, in exchange for campaign funds. I believe it is impossible to win a presidential election today without Illuminati support. The Kennedy family was "punished" because they tried to disobey them. The Kennedys were independent-minded and too difficult to "control.

Officially, the United Nations' mission is to work for world peace. It wants to perform both peacekeeping and military domination functions. Giving this role to the UN should reduce the military power of nations, and encourage them to depend more and more on outside or international organizations. They will thus offer less resistance when the Illuminati takeover occurs.

I was told that the New World Order would be officially revealed before the year 2020. But this may be just propaganda from the Illuminati, because they keep changing the dates. I personally believe that the Illuminati will openly reveal themselves before the middle of this century. But this is just a personal opinion.

Question: What is the Illuminati's plan for the Middle East and what will be the consequences for the rest of the world? Will we see a third world war?

Answer: The Middle East conflict is all about benefiting the Illuminati. They hate Israel. They hope that one day Israel will be destroyed, and are biding their time. They will use the United Nations to propose a plan for peace in the Middle East, which will be welcomed by many.

But, at the same time, it is the Illuminati who secretly arm the warring parties, to maintain the conflict. They are people full of duplicity. For example, in the past they used the USSR to smuggle weapons into Palestine in the name of "friendship" between the USSR and the Arab nations. Meanwhile, the American Illuminati have smuggled weapons into Israel for similar reasons.

The Illuminati love to play chess. They maintain wars between nations to bring out a new order from chaos. Russia will become powerful again. It is too strong militarily to accept to be reduced to a secondary role. All the Illuminati who were military trainers went to Russia to be trained there themselves. In the New World Order, the Russians will be stronger and better placed than the Americans.

You want to know what the endgame is going to be, as the Illuminati taught me. It was propaganda, but here's how they believe the New World Order is going to be set up: There's going to be ongoing conflict in the Middle East. These hostilities will culminate in a serious threat of nuclear war.

There is going to be an economic collapse in the U.S. and Europe, just like in the Great Depression. One of the reasons our economy continues to limp along is because of the U.S. Federal Reserve's monetary manipulation, which artificially plays with interest rates. But, one day, that won't work anymore. Or it will be made to stop working, and the economic crisis will break out. All the creditors, starting with the government, will want to be paid. There will be massive bankruptcies.

Europe will stabilize first. Germany, France and Great Britain will have the strongest economies. This may come as a surprise to the latter country! These three countries will have the United Nations establish a single world currency. Japan will also do well, but its economy will be weakened.

International forces, under the flag of the UN, will be sent to various locations to prevent riots. The leaders of the Illuminati will reveal themselves. They will ask the people to pledge their loyal service in this time of chaos and devastation.

It's not a very pleasant plan, is it? I don't know the exact schedule of all these events, and I don't even want to try to find out. What I can tell you is that anyone who doesn't have debt, who doesn't owe the government or the banks anything, who doesn't have credit on their backs, and who can pretty much support themselves, those people will probably do better than the others. If I had money, I wouldn't invest in stocks. I would buy gold instead! Gold is going to be the strongest asset in the world again. Our dollars won't be worth much. Remember what happened after our Civil War. Our currency will be worth no more than the Confederate currency after their defeat!

Having said that, I admit that it could all be Illuminati propaganda, to scare us. Maybe none of this will happen. I sincerely hope so. I also firmly believe that God is able to hold back the hand of the wicked, and to take care of our nation, as well as other nations, if we turn to Him.

Question: Would you say that the Illuminati are racists, as a whole? I ask this question because it seems to me that their agenda is very much about white supremacy!

Answer: The Illuminati are racists. They like the "Aryan" type. They firmly believe that the "pure" and "intelligent" (by their own standards) will rule the world. Occasionally they sacrifice some members of ethnic minorities in their ceremonies. They strive to genetically create a "superior race" that will rule the world with their children and descendants. They also admire Plato's Republic and believe that they will succeed in establishing this Utopia with their New World Order. They believe that their intellectual elites will rule, and that the masses will follow their leaders like sheep. This is how they see the world. They think that the occultists who rule them are "enlightened" and intelligent, and that the ordinary people are "sheep" to be led by the nose.

Question: Why did they put a black man in charge of the United Nations?

Answer: Because, for the moment, it serves their plans. They are liars. They are willing to give a prominent role to a popular figure to enhance the image of the United Nations. They want to pass themselves off as a group that works for "racial harmony," "unity" and "peace.

Real leaders never allow themselves to reveal in public what they really think. The United Nations is just setting the stage for what is going to be put in place. It is not the UN that wields the real power in the world. The UN will be a relatively unimportant body when the New World Order is established. Those who wield the real power will then reveal themselves. The U.N. is currently only a means of getting world public opinion to accept the idea of a "world community" and a "united world. The UN is only a step in their program.

Question: Are they trying to limit the world population? I am thinking in particular of the AIDS epidemic in Africa. Could the Illuminati have caused this epidemic?

Answer: I have read reports that the Illuminati may have spread some deadly viruses. But I doubt that it was them who spread the AIDS virus. Why not? Because many of the Illuminati leaders are openly homosexuals and pedophiles, and they would have put themselves in danger, because this virus is quite common in the United States. Most of the leaders I knew were homosexuals. So was I. It's accepted as a lifestyle in these circles, and even encouraged.

When the Illuminati spread viruses, they are viruses that can be treated, so that the leaders can be protected in case of an epidemic. I know, however, that some Illuminati groups are developing bacteriological weapons to threaten people who refuse to accept the New World Order. This was sometimes discussed in meetings of leaders. I cannot say what stage these projects are at, because it has been several years since I left the Illuminati.

PART FOURTEEN

History and future of the Illuminati

Question: *I have received invitations in my e-mail from neo-Nazi groups. I have read through their literature. They cleverly claim, using historical "facts," that the Illuminati are just a Jewish conspiracy, and that Hitler had to fight them. We know what happened next. My question is simple: Is it a Jewish conspiracy?*

Answer: Absolutely not! In fact, Hitler and his ilk, especially Himmler and Goebbels, were high level Illuminati. The Illuminati are extremely racist. When I was a child, I was forced to play "concentration camp," both on our Virginia farm, and also in Europe, in isolated camps in Germany.

Historically, the Jews have fought occultism. We see in Deuteronomy and the Old Testament how God, through the Jewish people, strove to cleanse the land of Israel of all the occult groups that operated there, such as those who worshipped Baal, Astarte, and other Canaanite and Babylonian gods.

Since the Illuminati trace their origin to these fertility deities, they are inherently deeply opposed to Jews. I would never trust the literature of neo-Nazis or other extremist groups, because their views are based on racism and the notion of a superior race. These are things that the Illuminati are very committed to. So this neo-Nazi group was telling you lies. They thought you didn't know that Nazism was founded by the German Illuminati!

Question: *Obviously, this dream of man dominating the world is not new, historically. History is full of failed attempts to conquer the world and dominate people. How old is the Illuminati dream of a New World Order?*

Answer: The Illuminati themselves teach that they have existed for centuries and centuries, even since the time of the Romans, and that Alexander the Great was one of their "prototypes. Their modern prototype was Hitler. But the Illuminati, as we know them today, were founded in the 17th century, under the influence of Catholicism, i.e. the Knights Templar and the Rosicrucians. The idea of a New World Order began to spread in the early 18th century with the ideas of Weishaupt and others. They have been working toward their current goal since the mid-18th century.

Question: Do the Illuminati manipulate society using history, such as that of Egypt, Rome or the British Empire? How far back does the Illuminati history go, even if their actions had other forms than today?

Answer: The Illuminati themselves say that they trace their origins to Babylon, around 3900 BC. This is probably propaganda. They claim to be based on the secret doctrines of all ancient religions and on occult and esoteric practices. But they seem to be more directly descended from the Knights Templar, a medieval order of knights, as well as the Rosicrucians, whose foundation dates back to about the same time. I don't know how much "programming" was mixed in with what we were taught about the history of the sect when I was a child. Whether this is a historical truth, I cannot say. Therefore, I cannot be an objective source of information. Like everywhere else, the Illuminati tend to want to idealize their roots.

Question: Since they are so smart, the Illuminati must know that empires, like civilizations, have generally not lasted very long. Maybe 200 years on average. Was the end of all these empires natural, or was it planned? Were the Illuminati responsible for the fall of the empires? Did they intentionally destroy civilizations in order to create new ones, the better to extend their domination?

Answer: When I was a child, I was taught that the Illuminati advised and financed all the monarchs of ancient history, just as they do for those of modern history. They claim that they are the ones who have manipulated history for the past 2000 years. But I believe that people also have free will. No Illuminati can completely control human nature. They don't know exactly how people will behave.

I don't believe they have accomplished all that they claim to have accomplished. However, it is true that they have exerted a profound influence, especially in the last 200 years, on all the governments of the world, and on international life. I say this on the basis of what I myself have observed among them.

Question: *Svali, you said that the Illuminati are working hard to achieve their goal of a New World Order. They want to be the leaders of this new society. So when will the Illuminati consider that they have achieved their goals? What is their vision for this "glorious" new order? What kind of policy will they pursue? Will it be dictatorial, communist or democratic? Will their desire to control the world succeed?*

Answer: I was taught that in this New World Order, first of all, there would be a strongly dictatorial and militaristic government. That is why they are putting all their members through this intense military training, at all levels, to be able to impose their policies. Why? Because not everyone will welcome their "enlightened" dictatorship with open arms. They will have opponents.

They are training their army in crowd control techniques. There will be camps where they will send opponents. Think of Hitler's Germany, which was a prototype for the New World Order. The Supreme World Council will set up an extremely authoritarian, hierarchical and centralized government, as is their current organization.

In a second phase, they will set up a semi-Marxist government, close to the militaristic socialism of the USSR. Marx was an Illuminatus. What he wrote was dictated to him. Financial decisions will be made at the national and international levels. People will be asked to work for a reduced salary, for the glory of serving the New World Order. Depending on their loyalty and performance, they will receive other compensation, just as in Marxist and Leninist Russia.

Once opponents are silenced and subdued, the Illuminati believe they will no longer need to struggle to control the world. They will have it in their power! They will then implement "genetic selection" programs, so that only the brightest and best will be allowed to procreate. Those who are considered "genetic rejects" will be sterilized. They have the same ideas as Hitler in this area. It's sad, but that's what they teach. Children with occult abilities will be detected and given special training to develop those abilities. They are already doing it now, but in secret. Once they are in power, they will do it openly.

Question: *Do the Illuminati have natural enemies, predators, or competitors in their goal of world control?*

Answer: No. At least I don't know them. They know that there are other groups besides them, such as the modern-day Knights Templar, or the Oto (Ordo Templi Orientis, a Catholic secret society that works with the Knights Templar), groups that are involved in a host of occult and illegal activities like them. On some issues, these groups disagree with the Illuminati. But they generally get along very well, and they exchange information.

In my opinion, their only real enemies are true Christians and the Church, who oppose everything they do. Because they are based on an occult spirituality, the Illuminati despise anything Jewish or Christian (I'm talking about true Christians). They are their mortal enemies. For true Christians engage in spiritual warfare which greatly hinders their action.

Question: How do you view the role of China and Russia, in light of recent events, and based on what you knew when you were in the cult?

Answer: Russia will be the military base of the Illuminati, and the source of their power in this area. The Illuminati consider Russia's military leaders to be the best and most disciplined in the world. China will be considered a more important power than the United States, because it also has its roots in Eastern occultism. But the real power of the Illuminati will come from Europe. This is what I was taught in this group.

China will administer the East, and Russia the Northern Hemisphere. I tell you what I have learned. But never forget that there was some "programming" involved! One of my most difficult tasks since leaving the Illuminati has been to evaluate what was true in what I was taught and what was just idealism or propaganda. I am not an Illuminati expert. Don't consider me an authority on the subject. The position I held was not high at all. I was on the San Diego metropolitan area leadership council for several years, but I had few contacts internationally.

FIFTEENTH PART

Television, a perfect instrument of mental control

Question: Svali, what role does television play? You were a trainer and programmer for the Illuminati. What role did television play as an instrument of mind control? How does it work on the brain? Why is television the perfect instrument for mind control of the masses? Give us some details.

Answer: It is important to understand that when we watch television, the brain begins to emit "alpha" waves, which are the waves of relaxation and rest. In this mental state, we are highly susceptible to suggestion. Have you ever noticed the glassy eyes of those who have just watched television for a while? This is due to the fact that one has been in an alpha wave state for a long time, in a mental state that is close to split personality. And again, I'm only talking about people who have not been raised under Illuminati mind control!

Remember also all those studies that showed, a few years ago, that "violence on television does not affect children's behavior". Guess who funded them! They are a bunch of liars. There is no doubt that what children watch on television does affect their behavior. The Illuminati psychologists know this! They knowingly use television to influence "the masses". They can't completely change the personality of most citizens, but they can desensitize them to an increasing acceptance of violence, pornography and the occult, while influencing the perceptions of young children.

Most cartoons carry a subtle message, as well as subliminal messages, designed to influence the next generation, as well as to destroy family values and traditional morality, making them seem outdated and "politically incorrect. Television today has a profound influence on our society, especially on young children. How many parents have allowed television to be their children's "babysitter" while having no idea what their children are watching?

I am sometimes horrified to hear my 12-year-old son tell me about the movies his classmates have watched on television, movies that depict mass murder, violence, and occult horrors. I would never allow impressionable children to watch movies like The Matrix, Fight Club, or the new Exorcist, for example, or like the movies that some teenagers love so much.

The Illuminati also play with sounds and images. They use image bombardment, as seen on many modern advertisements. Some television shows glorify the occult outright, or feature young, pretty witches, vampires and shape-shifting wizards.

Question: *Name the major Illuminati-inspired programs on television, or those that promote Illuminati ideas. What are their characteristics?*

Answer: The media is so infiltrated that one should ask what shows do not carry their ideas! Look at the Saturday morning cartoons, filled with occultism and witchcraft, which glorify paganism, or the movies that openly use mind control techniques. Look at most video games, which show scenes of "mental programming" with torture. I was very saddened to see this. The hero had to "save" the victim before he was tortured to death...

I would say that 90% of cartoons have occult themes, designed to capture the attention of children. This is how they are subtly indoctrinated to accept spirit "guides" or animal "guides", or to get used to occult training techniques. Even the "cute" little Pokémon, those docile creatures, can become real demons, once their "trainer" has "programmed" them to change their personality. This is too much like what the Illuminati does to docile children to make me feel better!

Personally, I don't watch much television. Sometimes I watch geographical reports, or a comedy movie. But, in general, I avoid watching it. I've heard too many discussions in the Illuminati, in executive meetings, and with the group's psychologists, about how they use television to subtly influence the masses, without them even knowing it! So I chose not to be influenced. Compare the television shows of the 1950's to today's shows, and you will get a good idea of the moral decline of our society!

Question: *What about the influence of pop music? Is it also used as a means of mind control? I believe that Cathy O'Brien, a survivor of CIA* *methods, has accused country music and a number of singers of being involved in this mental manipulation, and points to Nashville, Tennessee, as the center of this manipulation.*

Answer: Country music is definitely influenced, but it's mostly rock music that is controlled by the Illuminati. I once watched a rock show and couldn't believe what I was seeing! I couldn't believe it! Some rockers have butterfly tattoos all over their bodies (the butterfly is a sign of the mind control method called Monarch). I heard one singing, "Come on, butterfly... Let's run away to a better world...!"

This song was filled with "programmer" symbols. I believe that Britney Spears, Eminem, and other singers are used by the Illuminati to sing songs that people like. Some of them have a neo-Nazi look and carry hateful lyrics. This is no accident. In fact, many of the top pop singers are former fellows of the "Mickey Mouse Club," another branch of good old Illuminatus Walt Disney's empire! I believe they were offered star status, in exchange for their submission, or their acceptance of being used to mentally control the population.

How many songs praise suicide, violence, despair, or New Age spirituality in pop and rock music today! Take the trouble to read the lyrics of these songs! (But I ask the survivors of mind control to be careful, and not to let certain lyrics trigger "programmed" reactions in them!)

Question: What can be done to repair the damage already done by television and music?

Answer: Stop looking at it or listening to it! But that's easier said than done! However, when you stop watching or listening, the reinforcement of the conditioning stops. But how many people are completely addicted to their "TV moment"! I also believe that one of the best ways to repair the damage done is to replace negative or misleading messages with the truth. I do a daily study of God's Word to "renew my mind," as the epistle to the Romans puts it. I find this study infinitely more invigorating and rejuvenating than anything offered on television or radio!

Question: Svali, I'm sure you remember a few years ago that some Japanese cartoons, such as Pokémon, caused hundreds of children to have epileptic fits. Did the makers of these films not know this at the beginning, or was it a test of mind control of the population? Are the Illuminati programmers aware of this? Are they doing it to control the population? What do you think?

Answer: I don't know if it was intentional or not, since it happened after I left the Illuminati. I had never heard of it. But I can tell you that I never let my son watch Pokémon, even when he tells me that "all his friends watch them. I believe that these cartoons have a strong occult connotation. Just look at the Pokémon's eyes turn "red" when they change personality. This is similar to what happens to people who have been mind-controlled by demons.

I can't stand these movies, despite their popularity. I am very sad to see the effect they have on children. I would like to recall the alpha wave effect, to say that children are totally "immersed" in these movies.

Have you ever watched young children watching cartoons like this? Their eyes become glassy, their jaws drop, they become completely passive, and even their breathing slows down. It is for these reasons that I am not a fan of TV at all, especially because of its effects on young children. How many of them have learned to laugh at gratuitous violence, and find it "funny"! I even know of a very popular TV show that shows young people abusing their parents and filming it "just for fun"!

Question: I am reading an article that will probably interest you: From April 20, 2001:

"The hit discovered in Pokémon cartoons! Psychologists in the Russian city of Krasnodar have asked the Russian government to ban Pokémon cartoons from television. These cartoons had already been broadcasted on the national state channel ORT. They recalled that these films had already been banned in many countries, including Japan itself. Psychologists in Krasnodar claim that the "stroke system" is applied in these films, and that it negatively affects the subconscious of children. This system introduces a real "neurolinguistic programming". The children become like "zombies". Psychologists speak of "intellectual genocide". According to them, these cartoons encourage cruelty and aggressiveness, and the clothes of the heroes have many signs symbolizing death.

Answer: I don't know exactly what this "move system" is, but it seems obvious to me that the Russians have detected a subliminal method of mind control that has negative effects on children. I am not surprised. I have already said what I think about Pokémon. I also know of another card game that is even worse, called Magicke. Don't forget the role-playing games that mesmerize kids, like Dungeons and Dragons Online, Diablo, and so many others. The list is long!

PART SIXTEEN

The "lone murderers"

American Editor's Note: Warning! This section includes some pretty raw descriptions of the "programming" methods of the killers, and the brutal torture of children by the Illuminati. Svali asked me to publish her story, and I decided not to change anything in her account.

Question: Svali, you've heard of these "lone assassins," such as Timothy Mcveigh (the Oklahoma City killer), Lee Harvey Oswald (President Kennedy's assassin), Sirhan Sirhan (Robert Kennedy's assassin), John Hinkley (who made an assassination attempt on President Reagan), Eric Harris and Dylan Klebold (the Columbine High School killers). I'm sure you could name a few more. What do you think? Many of these killers have ties to the military, either directly or through their families. They are said to be mind control slaves. It was even said that Mcveigh had a microchip implanted in his body.

Is it possible that these men were mind control slaves? Can you tell us how easy it is to program these mind control slaves? How are they programmed? What are the signs that could show you that these criminals could have been "programmed"?

Answer: I am quite sure that some of these killers have gone through MK ULTRA type of mind programming. They may have been victims of military mind control programs and "gone bad". In fact, I know that some of these henchmen did. If you read their histories, you will see that they are almost always associated with Nazi or occult groups, and that Nazi symbols have often been found on them.

Why am I convinced that they were mentally programmed? First of all, because these men didn't just decide one day to pick up a gun and kill. They had to learn how to aim and shoot in a safe way. Where did they receive this training? Where did they develop their killing skills?

When I was a trainer with the Illuminati, there was an order that the trainers had to learn to use first, before working with their subjects. You should know that in the Illuminati, ALL children are trained to be assassins. I have been through this training myself, and I have never known a child in the Illuminati who has not. What is this order? The command "Halt" is the first command that is given to future assassins, whether they are children or adults. They are programmed to stop dead, to freeze in place, as soon as they hear the command "Halt!

Why do instructors have to teach their students to obey this order? Because they run the real risk of being killed by their students. The programming of this command "Halt" completely controls any desire for revenge. Since their childhood, these people have been subjected to all sorts of atrocious tortures aimed at teaching them to obey without question. From the age of five, they are taught to shoot, first with air guns and then with real guns. They are also trained with computer equipment that simulates reality (virtual reality programs).

These are people who are trained from early childhood to kill coldly, without showing the slightest emotion. In these computerized simulations, they are ordered to kill their own brother or sister. Since they are also under hypnosis at the time, they are convinced that this is reality. This is how their obedience is tested. They put my son through this horrible training. He cried as he told me how horribly anxious he was the next day, thinking he had killed his sister. He almost died of shock when he saw her alive. If he had not seen her, he would have been completely convinced that he had killed her in the simulation!

After being tortured, abused and raped all their lives, these poor victims feel a terrible rage against their torturers, who develop this hatred in them to make them better murderers. These people are thus trained and programmed to eliminate the "enemies" and the "weak" at the first commandment, for the good of the "family" and for their own glory. But sometimes these children or adults in "training" become difficult to control, because of the intense hatred that drives them.

I have known trainers who were killed by some of their "students" during the night, because they went too far, or did not protect themselves sufficiently. This was considered one of the "hazards of the job". I was always very careful. Every instructor knows that during the night, some students can get out of control. It always happens. These rebels were then very severely punished, imprisoned for several days and tortured, so as to teach them how to behave. Those who became particularly disturbed and unstable could end up being considered "unrecoverable" and eliminated. They could also be sent to a mental asylum, where no one believed their "paranoid delusions" when they said they were being "taught to murder.

As a result, trainers who were too brutal sometimes had difficulty controlling their students, and some ended up being murdered. These "accidents" were carefully covered up. Now you can see why the FBI does little to shut down websites that glorify the occult, or to investigate those accused of belonging to an organized occult group!

People don't just become murderers. They have been carefully and gradually taught to overcome the horror that one naturally feels when one kills another human being. This learning process begins in childhood with the Illuminati. They force children to learn to kill.

This is how they do it. This is how they did it to me: They take a two-year-old child, and put him in a metal cage connected to electrodes. They give him severe electric shocks. They take him out of the cage, and put a kitten in his hands. Then they order him to wring the kitten's neck. The child cries and usually refuses. They put the child back in the cage, and electrocute him until the child almost loses consciousness. They take the child out of the cage again, and again order him to kill the kitten. The child will start shaking all over and crying, but he will kill the kitten, because he is afraid of the torture. Then he will go and vomit in a corner, while the adult congratulates him for having "done a good job".

This is only the first step. The child is then given larger and larger animals to kill as they grow. Then they are ordered to kill a baby, either in a "virtual reality exercise" or in real life. By the age of nine, these children know how to cock a gun, aim, and shoot at a target, as soon as they are ordered. They are then trained with dummies that perfectly imitate human beings. Then with animals. Then with men, usually "irrecoverable" ones. They are also trained on virtual reality simulation programs. If they do a "good job", they are highly rewarded. But they are tortured if they refuse to obey.

The older the children get, the more they are trained. Before the age of 15, most of these children are forced to fight each other in the presence of spectators. High-level Illuminati come to watch these "games," just as in the days of the ancient gladiators. These fights rarely end in death. They stop when one of the children is defeated and knocked down. They use every weapon imaginable, and must learn to fight for their lives. If a child loses a fight, he is severely punished by his trainer, because he has "lost face". If he wins, he is rewarded for his "strength" and "skill" in handling weapons.

By the time they reach the age of 21, these young people have become real killing machines. They have been given a whole set of coded messages, and they are constantly tested to see if they will obey the first order. This is how the children of the German Illuminati are raised. I had to go through this training myself.

Question: Svali, you have already told us that learning the command "Halt! What exactly is this command? Is it just a code word, or is it something more complicated?

Answer: Normally, this command consists of a code that completely paralyzes the child or adult so programmed. It is usually a short series of numbers, such as "354!" That's just one example, it's not that exact code! Or, it's a German word followed by a combination of numbers.

All children try to get back at their trainers. This always happens when they are young. They are then severely punished, imprisoned and isolated, even beaten and electrocuted, to teach them not to do this anymore.

They are then taught the command "Halt!" under hypnosis, after having been drugged and subjected to extreme trauma. They are taught to react instantly to the command and to bring their bodies to a complete stop. They are told that if they don't, they will be tortured as punishment. This learning is often reinforced.

PART SEVENTEEN

The work of trainers and programmers

Question: Svali, can you tell us about the incredible properties of the human brain? What is your experience with this subject when you were a member of the Illuminati? I believe that photographic visual memory is only one of these properties.

Answer: Research has proven that we only use a small portion of our brain's capabilities. The Illuminati and other similar groups know this. That is why they have developed their training and stimulation programs to encourage children to use their normally unused brainpower.

In a hypnotic trance state, the human brain has been found to be capable of photographic memory. A person under hypnosis is able to remember events completely in their smallest details. The brain never loses anything. In our conscious life, we simply use "filters" to manage the information that comes to us. Otherwise our senses would be too bombarded, and we would be constantly distracted.

A hypnotic induction can remove all of these filters as a suggestion is implanted in the brain. The person can then "download" all the information contained in his or her memory and transmit it to the trainer.

Other abilities that are developed include: learning foreign languages (Illuminati children are taught from two to five languages, and even more, depending on their abilities); physical strength (these children have greater physical strength than other children of their age); occult abilities (these are highly sought after, and developed to the maximum).

This is how children learn telekinesis (moving objects by the "power of thought"), divination and the ability to obtain all kinds of information about others, the ability to travel through time, or in other spiritual dimensions, the ability to kill an animal or a man by the "power of thought", without even touching them, or astral travel (going out of the body in spirit). Children can thus leave their bodies in spirit, enter a room while being invisible, describe what it contains, listen to conversations, etc.

Children's intellectual capacities are also developed. Their average IQ can reach at least 120, up to 200 and above. IQs of 160 and above are common among the Illuminati. The particular skills that are developed depend on the child's or adult's future role in the group.

Question: Svali, you are probably familiar with the current TV series called "The Pretender". After what you have just said, I understand better the objectives of this series! Perhaps it is inspired by the techniques of mental programming or the history of the Illuminati?

Answer: I have never watched this series, because when I tried to do so a few years ago, the first two minutes triggered too many "programmed reactions" in me. I had to get up and leave the room. Later, I said to my husband, "I can't believe they are showing this openly on TV!" Yes, this series is directly inspired by mental programming techniques. But in our society, which is used to denying everything, this is considered "fiction. The only people who know it's true are those who had to undergo this programming!

Question: Could these mental programming techniques be used to develop our intellectual capacities, but without us losing control of our brain? A few years ago there was a lot of talk about so-called "mental machines", involving virtual reality headsets. What do you know about this? Do these machines produce results?

Answer: I'm sorry, but I don't know of any mental programming method that produces "good" results. Why not? Because most of these methods are traumatic. But even if they weren't, such machines and methods, if they fell into the wrong hands, would still be used to control and dominate others. In all these methods, there is someone programming the brains of others, and someone being programmed. Most of these "mental machines" and virtual reality headsets do not produce very good results. In order for them to work well, the subjects trained would have to be young, and they would also have to be heavily traumatized. It's sad, but it's true.

Furthermore, most of the abilities that are developed in the Illuminati are dangerous and destructive. The ability to travel through time and space is very costly to the human body. People who use this ability too often destroy their health, or shorten their life span considerably. I have known Illuminati, in the "spiritual" field, who practiced this. But they had completely white hair by the age of 22! Most of these people age very quickly, because their organism and their psyche are destroyed. The Illuminati themselves know this and avoid using these faculties too much.

It is important to know that it is the demons that make it possible to develop these faculties. Some people who have practiced these things have even ended up going crazy. I would certainly not recommend anyone to try to develop these faculties, to anyone, because it would be playing with fire. It is a very dangerous weapon! That's why I absolutely refuse to touch these things. This is one of the reasons why, a few years ago, I closed all these spiritual doors in my life, and I gave up these occult abilities. Now I can't do divination on people, or astral travel, or even speak five languages! I am so happy that I can't do all that anymore! Because my life belongs to Jesus, and that is a hundred times better for me! It develops my spiritual life much better than all these methods!

Question: Can you tell us more about these occult abilities, such as telepathy, telekinesis, or time travel? How do the Illuminati use these abilities?

Answer: First of all, it is important to understand that time travelers are often in a different state of consciousness than their normal state. They leave their bodies in spirit, and travel backwards in time on a spiritual level. I have personally found that those who do this time travel are in a sort of deep coma. Their breathing and heart rate slow down, their skin becomes pale and cold. It is also necessary to start by making a sacrifice to "open the portal". The first few times, the one who makes this kind of journey almost always has to be accompanied by a guide, to lead them and help them back. It was always something very scary, because you could "get lost" and never come back to the present!

I used to hate it. I now believe that it is demons that allow this to happen. Because it is something that the Bible forbids. That's one of the reasons why I don't like to remember it. These time travels were almost always in the past. There was some kind of barrier that prevented us from traveling into the future. You could only travel into the future for a period of a day or two. I don't know why there was this barrier.

But there were no barriers to visiting the past. The Illuminati travel to the past for several reasons. First, to learn about history, to seek advice and counsel from some of the great personalities who lived in the past, and to prove to others the "glorious" historical continuity of the Illuminati. I have seen occult ceremonies that took place at Stonehenge 1000 years ago, and visited the courts of monarchies that practiced these rites. I now believe that it was all a seduction, a lie organized by demons. None of the "historical" information obtained by this means can be trusted.

Time travel was only allowed for short periods of time. The Illuminati forbade doing so for longer periods of time because of the health and psychological problems caused by such "travel. These things are extremely destructive.

Question: *Can these methods be used to influence people, e.g. politicians, businessmen, military leaders, etc., or to inject thoughts into them?*

Answer: Not that I know of. There is a limit to the use of these methods. It was much more effective for us to blackmail these people, or to bribe them. I think that the effectiveness of these occult phenomena is sometimes overestimated, because people have free will, except those who are directly controlled by the Illuminati.

Question: *How much can they change the collective consciousness of the world, especially by practicing time travel? How many people would have to practice these techniques to achieve this goal?*

Answer: They are not trying to do that. Remember that God is in control of history, not the Illuminati or any other group.

Question: *Do the Illuminati have any kind of specialists in these methods, or people who are employed full time in this area?*

Answer: They have people who do this more often than others. These are the ones who are in the "spiritual" field, and who specialize in these "spiritual" techniques, instead of specializing in science, education or military affairs. These people always age faster than others, and they quickly get gray hair. They themselves must limit the use of these techniques, which are so destructive.

Some of these methods are also practiced in the context of "theta programming", which concerns the programming of everything occult. Remember in the movie The Matrix, those children who learn to bend spoons by the "power of thought"! This is pure "theta programming", and I was horrified to see it. Hollywood is running the show! These faculties are used to learn how to "kill with thought".

I have seen animals killed in this way, by a group of people gathered in a circle around the animal, "focusing" on it. They are supposed to be able to kill people this way too. They can also listen or see from a distance.

It is not at all a "new dimension" or an "innate ability of the human body" that should be discovered. It is actually demons influencing people and revealing their knowledge to them. But this always ends up destroying those who practice these things intensively. Demons want to destroy the human race, because they know that God loves man. Demons hate God and man, because we are His beloved creation.

The Bible talks about all these occult techniques, like astral travel or time travel. The Bible calls these things witchcraft and spiritualism. God forbids us to practice these things for a good reason: to protect ourselves. I have heard of people who never came back from these "trips", who died, or who went crazy after practicing these things. I would never advise anyone to get involved in this field, when life on this earth is full of good things that are not destructive.

I am so glad I don't have to witness or practice such things anymore! I have forever renounced all this in my life. I have closed all doors to demons and their activity. I have also lost all my abilities in this area, and that is a great relief to me!

PART EIGHTEEN

Readers' questions (1)

Question: Do the Illuminati families trace their origins to particular European cities?

Answer: Yes, but it depends on the family. There is the German branch, the French branch, the English branch, and the Russian branch. Each branch has its roots in certain cities and regions of Europe. The cities of central Germany and Austria are the cradles of the German branch. This branch can be traced back to the Knights Templar, who unified the European nations at the time of the Crusades.

Question: Do the Illuminati believe in God? Do they consider Him a liar?

Answer: The Illuminati believe in the deification of man through knowledge. They know that there are supernatural beings who help them in this process. But they do not necessarily divide these supernatural beings into "good" and "evil. Rather, they speak of those who are "enlightened" and those who are "entranced." They believe in the existence of the God of Christians. But they think that Christians are not "enlightened" and that they do not have the "big picture" that they have. They think that Christians are sheep who have "swallowed" a nice story to make them feel better, because they are "too weak" to know "the whole truth". This is how the Illuminati would talk to you. They tend to be cynical about the God of Christians. They think he is just a "placebo" for the weak!

Question: Do they consider their god to be a liar too, even if he lies "for the good"? How can they trust their god?

Answer: They believe in many gods. Indeed, they believe that their "gods" are liars. These gods are able to give them power, wealth, glory, and everything they desire. But they know that they have to pay a price for all this, a horrible price. They say that you don't get something for nothing, and that the more they have to pay, the more valuable what they get is. It's hard to explain this kind of thinking to those who are not Illuminati. Most people think they are just horrible Satanists, enemies of Christianity. They don't see themselves that way. They do mock and despise Christians, but only because they want their followers to understand that it is Christians who are "seduced. It is Satan, the "god of this world," who has blinded them. So the Illuminati do not trust their gods any more than they trust any other person.

Remember that trust does not exist in them. They are taught from childhood that "betrayal is the ultimate ideal"! If you were to ask them if they trust their gods, they would look at you with a surprised look, and say, "You have to be an idiot to trust what you don't know!"

Question: *Do they consider the God of Christians as a God filled with naive love?*

Answer: Yes, yes! They think he is very naive, and that he is leading his followers to disaster. Do you understand the extent of their arrogance?

Question: *if they torture and terrorize those they love who are of a lower rank, what difference do they make between love and hate?*

Answer: They don't know the difference between love and hate. When they torture their own children, they tell them, "I am doing this because I love you!" For them, the greatest proof of love is to make their children strong, capable of leading and advancing in the group, by any means possible.

If a leader spots a girl and wants to turn her into a prostitute, the girl's parents will be very happy to give her to him, because they know that she will reach a "better" position in the group. At the same time, they continue to teach their children that "betrayal is the highest ideal" and that no one should ever be trusted!

I remember suffering hundreds of betrayals. They would say to me when I was suffering, "This is what is in the heart of man! They thought they were teaching me something very important that would help me in life. In a way, they were right, because everyone in that group is evil and vicious. Those who are naive are mercilessly trampled and hurt. I have known a few parents who wanted to spare their children from certain harsh "trainings" because they loved them. But they were often ruthlessly dismissed by the ruling families, who considered these parents as "weak", incapable of teaching their children properly.

Question: *Could you tell us a little more about their religious beliefs? Do they believe in reincarnation? Heaven and Hell? In sin and forgiveness of sins?*

Answer: The Illuminati have many religious beliefs. There are those who are followers of Druidism, those who are Rosicrucians, those who practice the Babylonian or Egyptian mysteries, and those who practice the occult. Children must learn all these things in the course of their training.

The Illuminati believe that they have succeeded in choosing the best of all these religions and synthesizing them. So there is not just one religion among the Illuminati. In Washington, D.C., the main trainers were druids, as well as those who followed Babylonian traditions. In San Diego, they practiced more of the Egyptian mysteries, partly because Colonel Aquinos was the leader of that group, and he was a follower of the Temple of Set.

What I am telling you is just a brief statement. They believe that reincarnation is possible, because of the time travel they do, but they do not emphasize it in their teachings. They believe that there will be a "final sphere" of "white light. This represents for them a "complete enlightenment". This is their concept of Paradise. They believe that they are protected from Hell because they are the only ones who are "enlightened. Hell, for them, is reserved for those who are not "enlightened" like them, for those who are still "in darkness". Their concept of Hell is therefore different from that of the Bible. For them, Hell is to remain forever in an inferior spiritual situation, without ever being able to reach enlightenment in the afterlife. They also believe that there are different levels of spiritual development after death, depending on the progress they have made on earth.

For them, sin is being weak and stupid. It is not to use the hidden capacities in man. It means not being able to progress. I have never heard of "forgiveness of sins". If you fail, you must be punished or put to death. It is simple. Members of the Druidic branch also believe in the existence of elves and elemental spirits. They believe that life exists in all areas of creation.

Question: *Some researchers believe that the Illuminati have the general population ingest substances or things designed to weaken their enemies. Do you know if the Illuminati are advising their members to avoid, for example: additives mixed into water and food products, vaccines, certain drugs, tampered food products, microwaved food, implants, certain dental preparations, and certain radiation or chemicals?*

Answer: In general, leaders are protected from all of the things you just named. They are instructed never to drink or take drugs or harmful products. They don't go so far as to avoid certain foods or microwaved foods. They don't worry about that. But, at their meetings, healthy food is served, and they know the importance of good nutrition.

They don't put their higher-ups through all their mental programming experiments because of the risks involved. These adults and their children have to go through special programs that are different from the programs designed for the lower levels. They get vaccinations. But even when their children get sick, they go to a healer. They also take medicine when they need it, such as antibiotics, etc.

Question: *Some believe that Mormons, Jehovah's Witnesses, pagans, New Agers, Satanists, and even charismatics all belong to religions or movements created by the same occult schemers. Are these groups, or at least their leaders, considered allies by the Illuminati?*

Some of these groups are secretly affiliated with the Illuminati because of the money they may have received from them, or because of some free "training" they may have received. Others are simply sympathizers. The Mormons became affiliated with the Illuminati in the 1950s. So did the Jehovah's Witnesses. I have never heard of Charismatics or Pagans affiliating. Pagans are considered "amateurs" by the Illuminati. New Age people and Satanists are sympathizers.

Question: *Do they respect Science or History, considering that it strengthens them in their own beliefs?*

Answer: No. They respect science, but they try to rewrite history in their own way. They make plays for their children, to make them understand "real" History. They also practice time travel, but I don't trust the "historical" information obtained by this means, because I believe that it is a demonic seduction.

The Illuminati teach their children that powerful Illuminati have been secretly advising all the monarchs of Europe, and indeed all the monarchs of the earth, since the beginning of history. Is this true, or is it propaganda? I don't know. They also tell their children that there is, under the site of Stonehenge, a large room filled with the skeletons of people offered in sacrifice. Reality or fiction? I don't know, and I can't finance an archaeological expedition that could verify it!

I therefore doubt the veracity of their teachings, since they exclude the role of faith in God, and deny His ability to repel evil. For my part, I believe that it is God, and not the evil one, who has always controlled human history.

PART NINETEEN

Readers' questions (2)

Question: I am very concerned about the New World Order plan, and I would like to know if there are any possible ways to prevent the Illuminati from carrying out this plan.

Answer: I know I sound cynical, but I wish you luck! I sincerely hope you make it! I think it would take a lot of people coming together to stop them, and a lot of money and great lawyers!

Personally, I don't know of any group that is actually working to stop them. I live in a rural area, and I have no such contacts. I would love to see Christians dedicated to stopping the horrible torture of little children, and I would be willing to pray for them. But this is also a spiritual battle. Everyone who is involved in these occult issues needs to be well aware of this spiritual battle. The Illuminati are also fighting on a spiritual level. Anyone who would want to stop them without prayer would be very vulnerable, in my opinion.

Question: Have you considered a plan similar to Alcoholics Anonymous to help victims of ritual abuse recover? My personal experience has shown me that such a plan can work, as long as it is spiritual.

Response: I believe that similar groups already exist. They already deal with incest victims, and many have addressed the issue of ritual abuse. I told you, I live in a rural area. My village has a population of 100 people, including squirrels and cows! I couldn't really help groups that deal with ritual abuse. These groups are usually located in large metropolitan areas. In fact, I myself have to drive two hours every month to attend therapy. I couldn't get one closer to home!

Question: Could you read anything you wanted to when you were in the Illuminati? Were there things you were not allowed to read? If nothing is forbidden, some of the Illuminati may find that they are being told lies...

Answer: No, you are wrong. I could read anything I wanted. You have to understand the Illuminati mindset. When I was little, my parents told me that everyone was secretly part of the Illuminati, and that people's apparent behavior was just a facade.

When they took me to a friend's house for dinner and performed an occult ceremony at the end of the meal, I thought everyone was doing the same. I had always believed, since I was a child, that everyone did that. I could see that some books talked about love, tenderness and trust. But I thought it was all an act, and that the people who wrote these books were not inspired by reality.

So I was living in two completely different worlds: the "day" world and the "night" world! To question something, you have to start by taking a certain distance. I had never reached such a maturity. I had no reason to question their teachings. I didn't start doing that until I became an adult. Think about that. Also, our society was filled with movies and television shows that only reinforced what the Illuminati were teaching us, starting with Walt Disney movies. I listened to "heavy metal" rock bands, and their values were what I was being taught. In fact, outside of Christian books, there isn't much in this world that teaches us to trust others!

Question: I was shocked to learn that you were forced to suppress or kill one of your friends. Are many Illuminati forced to do this during their training, or is it reserved for punishment? Is it only strangers who are killed in this way? Can you talk about this, or is it too difficult for you?

Answer: This friend was also a member of the Illuminati. But she had been declared "unrecoverable. In the Illuminati, people are classified into only two groups: those who are "useful" and those who are "irredeemable. Everyone works very hard to be useful! This is not a common punishment, however. In fact, this kind of situation is quite rare. But my mother was a very ambitious person.

She was a senior trainer, and held the "spiritual" chair of the Washington Area Regional Council. The other chairs were the Army Chair, the Government Chair, the Executive Chair, the Education Chair, and the Science Chair. The Army chair was occupied by my mother's supervisor at the Pentagon, where she worked. This man's code name was Ashtoth.

The Illuminati usually seek out their victims from outside the group, either to sacrifice them in their rituals or to kill them. For me, it was a lesson I was never to forget. This was the case, because I didn't make any friends after that! I didn't like anyone higher than me, and I had no desire to befriend anyone my mother considered "worthy" of the "leader" I was.

Sometimes, but rarely, during military exercises, the weak ones or those who were too far behind were removed, to teach the others a lesson. I saw it myself once. But the children of the main leaders were never cut off. Only the children of the members who were at the bottom of the ladder were suppressed.

Question: You said that you begged God every night to give you a better home. But you were angry with God because he didn't answer your prayers. Were your prayers to the true God, or to the god of the Illuminati? If it was the real God, where had you learned that there was a good God?

Answer: that's a great question! I didn't pray to the Illuminati Gods, because I knew they were cruel, sadistic and scary. I was praying to a good God whose existence I had learned about through reading, television, and also through the innate knowledge that all children have, of the existence of a good God, somewhere up there.

I had also had some experiences with angels. I was protected as a child during a horribly traumatic experience, and it made me think that good existed too. The Illuminati never tried to stop me from praying because they believed that "positive" spirituality gave hope and could prevent suicide.

In fact, I was forbidden to get too involved with the occult in my daily activities because of the increased risk of suicide. They believe in keeping a "balance" even in this area.

Question: You said that "Papa Brogan" was the only "nice" adult you knew as a child. Do you mean that he showed you affection? In what way?

Answer: Dr. Timothy Brogan was a professor at George Washington University. He was a specialist in neuropsychology, and one of the main trainers among the Illuminati in the area. He was also a close friend of Sidney Gottlieb, one of my mother's "friends.

He could be very kind, but also very cruel. He would take me on his lap, calling me his "little one," and he would praise me warmly when I "behaved well. He taught me to play chess, and read me pieces of literature. He told me that I was his "adopted daughter" and that he was proud of me. We would have intellectual discussions late into the night, and it was he who passed on his ideas about leadership styles and training. Not all Illuminati activities are cruel and inhumane. This man could show affection and love. I played with his children, who were older than me. He patiently answered my questions about science, geography and other topics. I was completely bonded to him, which made the torture and sexual abuse he did to me particularly unbearable.

Question: *You said that your personality was completely fragmented, with over 7,000 fragments and 16 internal systems. Do you mean that you had many personalities, each of which was not aware of the others? Did any of your personalities actually enjoy their existence?*

Answer: Yes, my personality was fragmented into multiple personalities. Most of the Illuminati I have known have had many different personalities. In fact, I believe that everyone has a personality that is more or less disassociated. Even our local and regional leaders, like Jonathan, would regularly have their personalities "tuned up" by a few "tune-up" and "programming" sessions. I used to call them for this. The biggest dissociation was between our "day" and "night" lives. Most of my night personalities could communicate with the other parts. The more "developed" parts of my personalities were communicating information to the less "developed" parts. I could tell that many of my personalities really enjoyed their existence. I had about 140 separate personalities, which handled all my daily activities, work, friends, and hobbies.

I didn't just have bad experiences, like with Dr. Brogan. Some people congratulated me and told me that I would have an important position in the New World Order. It is true that they told everyone! I was to serve as an intermediary between governments of different nations, because of my language and psychological skills. Many of my internal personalities were very proud of their skills and accomplishments, and they were very saddened when I left!

(We believe that all these different "personalities" that were acting inside Svali were actually the many demons that possessed her, due to her occult activities and the doors that had been opened to them. Svali was delivered from these demons when she confessed her sins to the Lord, and closed all the doors that had been opened to the demons through occultism and witchcraft.)

Question: *Are all Illuminati who are not Germans also racist Nazis and genocidal maniacs? If the leaders of all countries in the world are Illuminati, that means they belong to all races. Are the white Illuminati opposed to the black Illuminati?*

Answer: Not all Illuminati groups are as fanatically racist as the German Illuminati, although many are. These people are generally extremely racist. But they also have a lot of practical sense. They understand that they cannot dominate the world without the help and cooperation of races other than the white race. Those who are loyal to them among the other races are promoted to leading positions in their countries. But they are always supervised by the great leaders of the Illuminati (who are white).

Moreover, they do not have the same opinion of Orientals as of other non-white races. For Orientals have a long tradition of mysticism and occultism, as in Tibet. They also have a very ancient culture, and they are very intelligent. For this reason, the Eastern branches of the Illuminati are highly respected, even in Europe. But all Illuminati believe that the real seat of world government will be in Europe.

Even in countries where the majority is not white, the main leaders are very often white. For example, in South America, the main leaders are of white descent, or barely mixed. In Africa, many of the leaders are actually white, but in secret, although many black leaders have shown extreme loyalty to the Illuminati. The Illuminati use black people. But no blacks are allowed to hold leadership positions in the world. These positions are already held by whites.

That said, I believe that the racist and hateful policies of the Illuminati are extremely despicable. I used to argue with my leaders about this and other issues of racism.

I hope I have answered some of your questions.

WHO IS SVALI?

S vali is a former occultist, who was a trainer for the "Illuminati". She taught the members of this secret society the techniques of mind control. After converting to Jesus Christ, while remaining anonymous, she decided to reveal everything she knew about this network and the dangers of this Luciferian movement.

She was released from her group in San Diego at the age of 38. Svali disappeared from circulation in July 2006. Her website (www.suite101.com) was deleted and her phone line was cut. Some of the articles on her site are archived in PDF at this address: www.fichier-pdf.fr/2012/11/24/ritual-abuse/

In January 2006, 6 months before her death, she gave an exclusive radio interview to Greg Szymanski: www.dailymotion.com/video/xx76t4_svali_news

How the sect accomplishes the programming

This article, in correlation with those already written, is very difficult for me. Why? Because it addresses some of the things I am most ashamed of in life. I had become a cult programmer, or "trainer" as they used to say, and here I will share some of the things I have done or witnessed on occasion. I also went through this as a child, so this article is also autobiographical. An autobiography can be an opportunity to brag, to feel joy or pain. As for me, I find myself in the latter category, to say the least. But I hope with all my heart that sharing my pain will help others avoid it or help society understand a little better what survivors have gone through.

This article will by no means cover the entire subject. Cult programming is a complex subject, which would fill volumes and volumes if one were to get to the bottom of it. I will therefore only write from my own experience with the Illuminati, which is one of many groups operating today, and will only cover the techniques used in the Washington, DC and San Diego, California area. It is possible that other locations use different techniques.

This article is NOT a substitute for the advice of a qualified therapist and is intended to be informative only. If you are a survivor of cult abuse, please be aware that this article and the subject matter can be extremely triggering, and therefore protect yourself.

What is a cult training or programming of people? In previous articles, I have mentioned the goals:

➢ Earning money

➢ Keeping it secret

➢ Demonstrate unconditional loyalty to group members

Programming, or training, is a method the cult has found to ensure that these goals are accomplished. In the Illuminati, programmers are called "trainers" because they are led to believe that they are not abusing anyone, but are just "training" the next generation. The trainers actually think they are doing a good job, "strengthening" the children, helping them focus on their "potential.

Some of these methods have been practiced for hundreds, perhaps thousands of years. I will divide programming into 5 main categories and address each one separately:

1. Silence training

2. Strength training

3. Loyalty training

4. Training to function within the group

5. Training of the mind

The first category, training in silence, begins at an early age, often before the child can speak. This is accomplished in many ways, depending on the child and the trainer, and may include: Questioning the child after a ceremony to find out what he or she has seen and heard. The very young child who would talk about these "naughty things" is punished severely and brutally, and told that no, he has not seen these things. This is repeated at frequent intervals until the child learns to block out the ceremonies.

Often an alter will be created through abuse, this will be a "protector" or "guardian", whose job it will be to ensure that the child does not remember what he or she has seen. This protector is told that if the child remembers, he or she will then be punished brutally.

Another method is to shock the child into a deep hypnotic trance, where he is told that he will forget what he saw or heard, that it was just a "bad dream". The child WANTS to forget, and will very quickly agree.

Psychological torture can be used, locking him in a cage, abandoning him, hanging him over a bridge, and then "rescuing" him later and telling him that if he denounces, he will be punished again.

He can be made to watch a mock punishment or a real punishment or the death of a traitor who has "spoken out."

When I was 4 years old, I was forced to watch a woman being flayed alive. Her crime: she had told "family business" to an outsider. Talking to outsiders is considered one of the worst crimes or betrayals a person can commit. The "death of a traitor" is one of the worst things imaginable in its horror and ranges from being crucified upside down to other equally gruesome scenarios.

Young children do not forget what they have seen and they become convinced that remaining silent is the safest way to stay alive.

This is done to ensure that the young child will not disclose the criminal activities they are witnessing during group activities, or even as an adult, when they are more actively involved in them.

Another staged story is frequently used: the "no one will believe your story" story (this is usually practiced with school children). The child is told over and over again that even if he or she reveals something, no one will believe it. The child is taken to a psychiatric hospital where he or she is briefly introduced to an inmate. The child is later told that people who speak out are considered "crazy" and sent to institutes, where they are severely punished and can never leave. These lies are told to further reinforce the importance of silence.

Another scenario may be that "everyone is participating". The child is told that in reality everyone is secretly part of the group, but that people are just pretending during the day. The child will be taken to a group member's house for dinner, where everyone is acting normally, and then a ritual or ceremony will follow. The child will then believe that there is no way out, since everyone is part of the group. Since most of the adults close to his parents are part of the group, he has no reason to question what he has been told.

The staging and psychological conditioning to forbid him to speak are infinite, with the only limits being the creativity of the adults around him.

Strength training

This type of training will also begin at a very young age, often as a baby. The child is subjected to a series of conditioning exercises whose goals are :

- ➢ Increase resistance to pain

- ➢ Increase physical fitness

- ➢ Increase the capacity of dissociation

- ➢ To force a quick memorization of objects (for school children)

- ➢ Creating fear and desire to please

These exercises may include: simulated military training, with "cops and prisoners" marches and games; shocking; physical abuse and torture; child and adult drugs; caging the child, where he or she is brutalized; deprivation of food, water, or sleep; abandonment for varying lengths of time; and being forced to witness brutality and abuse of others. The child is taught to remain completely silent during these displays or else is quickly and mercilessly punished for speaking out.

The scenes go on and on, the above is only a small part of the methods used.

Loyalty training

The third area of training has a large place in behavior. Loyalty involves agreement with the group, espousing its doctrines and beliefs. This training is sometimes more subtle, but it is also one of the most powerful influences on the group. The adults in the group model complete loyalty to their children. Escaping, leaving, or questioning the group's beliefs is rarely seen, and retaliation for questioning those in authority is swift and brutal. A person who questions the rightness of things or balks at doing his or her job can go back to being "re-trained," that is, shocked and tortured into submission.

But adults often find that the goals of the group are GOOD. They are convinced that they are helping the children, and during class the children are taught why these beliefs are good; they are told about the evolution of the group, where they will become the new leaders. There is a lot of discussion about when the group will "rule the world", to prove that they are in fact heralding a new order, when things will be "better for all".

Position and leadership are carrots at the end of the stick for group members to work harder and succeed. The rewards in the form of leadership and advancement are real and everyone tries to get ahead. Having a higher position means less abuse, being able to lead others and more control in a life that has had so little of that precious control. A play where a child is allowed to sit in a leader's seat and is told that one day he or she too will be in charge is often practiced to increase group loyalty. Award ceremonies, where those who work well are presented with badges, jewelry or other awards in front of everyone, are also frequently done.

A hard-working child who is a good performer receives praise and is allowed to join the adults for coffee or a meal, with the other children looking on enviously.

Children who progress through the system move up in rank, but an adult always has a higher rank than a young child. Now the growing child can direct younger children, tell them what to do, and even abuse them with adult approval. Being very young means being very abused and hurt for these groups; growing up actually gives the chance to vent the rage of being abused. The child begins to identify with the abusive adults, as they are less hurt, and is then invested in the identity of the abuser in the cult. This is strongly encouraged, as long as the act is not directed at members older or higher than the child or adolescent.

The child is imprisoned by becoming "one of them", he is "like them", and is associated with the group by his own guilt and shame, as well as by the need to vent his rage and pain with the permission of the group.

The child may experience ambivalence, but also extreme loyalty.

The group or trainer will also tell the child that they are the only ones who really know the child, having seen him/her act.

That they are the only ones who can see it and still love it, that no one loves them more than the "family".

The child is bombarded with messages that the group really does accept him/her, accepts them all, knowing the worst about him/her, in order to cement loyalty. The group uses sophisticated techniques based on behavioral psychology to ensure that it never even occurs to the child/teen/adult to leave the group.

Another form of loyalty programming is the "special program. This is one where the adults or trainer tell the child that they are "superior," or from a hidden royalty or a secret or adopted member of a high family line. The child may be told that he or she will be a world leader kept hidden for the moment, a special agent of the CIA, or a child prodigy who will lead when he or she is an adult. He may be told that there are very few like him; that no one else will be able to fulfill his extraordinary role; that he comes from a lineage that has continued for thousands of years! This is done to increase the child's loyalty to the group. If the child believes that all he has to do is simply wait today for his high, real position to be revealed to him one day, he will be more likely to develop loyalty to the group. This is one of the cruelest tricks the group plays on children, as they are deprived of normal love and attention, replaced by the false idea of being "special" or having a position. Very few survivors who have come out of these groups think of any inferiority; almost all believe for this reason that they are superior or that they were adopted, but that their real family is superior. I experienced this as well and as an adult, when I had to tell lies like this to children, I was disillusioned, this was one of the many reasons that I actually chose to leave. I could no longer stand to listen to other trainers and scientists laugh at the naivety of the people they were working with. I was once a child, eager to please and naive myself. I had believed the lies and it was a rude awakening to discover that I was NOT adopted from a royal line as I had been told. That I had been manipulated and deceived on purpose to increase my loyalty to the group!

Training for a job in the sect

The fourth category of training or programming is geared toward work within the cult.

Each person has a specific job assigned to them from early childhood in the Illuminati. The child is regularly tested during the early years for skills and abilities. The status of the parents as well as the child's intelligence and ability to dissociate will also play a role in the final job. Possible jobs in a cult are, but are not limited to: Those who clean up (after ceremonies, dramatizations) Those who take care of spiritual matters (leading conferences, priests or priestesses or acolytes) Those who punish (members who overstep the mark or make mistakes) Those who teach (the history of the cult, dead languages, historical lectures and dramatizations)

> ➢ The prostitutes

> ➢ The messengers

> ➢ The assassins

> ➢ The trainers

> ➢ Scientists (trained in behavioral science)

> ➢ Doctors, nurses, medical staff

> ➢ Military Leader (for military exercises)

The list can go on and on. The Illuminati is a complex group, with interchangeable roles. The length of training a child will need for their future adult role will often depend on the complexity of their final job. Sometimes the jobs overlap or one person will be trained for several jobs. A child raised around pornography may later learn how to operate a camera, for example. A nurse or doctor may also be in a training role or teach science. A person trained as a military leader will often also train as an assassin (MK-ULTRA).

These jobs are taught through conditioning principles from early childhood. The child is shown how the adult or teenager performs his or her role, i.e., a "model" of behavior. The child will also see the jobs done during their participation in the group. Once the role models are visualized, the child is told that he or she will be taught. The child is given clear instructions on what is expected of him/her. The work is broken down into steps and each step is carried out with a timeline. The child may be brutalized or tortured to create a "blank slate" or tabula rasa personality that will do whatever is asked. Behavior is then induced. If the child behaves well, he is praised and pampered. If not, they are severely punished. The child learns that it is much less painful to do what is asked of him. Then, once the behavior is learned, the trainer attaches the child with rewards, telling them how good they are and what a wonderful job they both do for the "family". The child is given the rewards and care he or she desperately craves and a trauma bond is created. One of the child's personality states WANTS to do well, there is a bond with the trainer or adult and he or she is constantly seeking approval. This bond will last throughout his or her adult life and we often see approval seeking personality states that remain in the beginning stage in an adult body.

Once the "work" is done, these states of perpetual approval-seeking will be demanded again from time to time. Another reward will be seen in the adult in the form of an advancement in status if he or she behaves well.

Spiritual formation

From the beginning, the Illuminati have been an intensely spiritual group. They worship ancient deities such as those of Babylon and Assyria (Baal and Astarot) and Egypt (Ra, Horus, Isis, etc.). They believe that the spiritual is the root of many of today's manifestations. It is for this reason that all children will undergo some form of spiritual training or programming. It is also to ensure their attachment to the group as well as to coerce or scare them into leaving.

Spiritual programming begins with the first ceremony of dedicating the child to a deity, even as early as the prenatal stage, when the fetus is dedicated in utero to a "heavenly mother" or other deity. The world of the small child will include visions of adults around him or her participating in ceremonies, and he or she will be forced to imitate the activities that were seen.

There may be baptisms with animal blood. There will be many consecrations and rites, including the transfer of family spirits to the young child, that of his mother, or father or grandfather. There may be some very frightening experiences. I don't want to argue here about the existence of the demon, but I would say that the group really believes it is real and that the manifestations seen during these rites are beyond anything that can be explained scientifically or rationally. When I was a child, I firmly believed in the reality of the demon as did all the adults around me.

Ceremonies will take place during which the demon is invoked and manifestations of his power, such as channeling, predictions or killing animals under mediumship. Using demonic abilities, objects moved by themselves or trees were thrown to the ground. Adults were involved in psychic power struggles, "readings" were done for people. And any training/programming session would invoke the demon to guide the trainer or infuse energy into the programming at hand. And often an invocation ceremony was done before a major programming session. The child was told that the demon was inside him and that if he tried to leave or mess up the programming, the demon would come and kill him. Any terrified child will believe this. There might be "bare hands surgery," where an "eye" would be injected into the abdomen and the child would be told that the eye could see him wherever he went and would denounce him if he tried to escape or question the group. Implants, thin metal rods, could be inserted to summon demonic forces. If the person tries to leave or stops the programming, the implants will cause intense pain.

The child will be forced to participate in the rites, which include the mutilation or killing of animals or even a baby.

There may be visits to woods or sacred places where statues of deities will be decorated with flowers and before the ritual participants will sing dressed in robes.

In some groups a specific program will orient the child against Christianity. Since Christianity is the antithesis of the Illuminati's occult practices, they often want their members to be unable to come in contact with the hope it would bring. Special sessions may include torturing the child. The child will often cry out for help or call out to God. At this point, the programmer will say to the child, "God has abandoned you, He couldn't love you, that's why you're hurting. If He were so powerful, He could stop this."

They will even ask the child to pray to God to stop it. The child will do this and then the trainer will hit the child even more. This will create a deep sense of despair in the child. He will truly believe that he has been abandoned by God, that he has remained deaf to his call. The child can be tortured or beaten when the name of Jesus is mentioned, to create a barrier to the mention of His name. Aversion can also be created through the use of hymns in sessions. Spiritual programming will cover a wide variety of areas. I have only briefly described a few of them.

This is only an overview of the cult's programming areas, especially those of the Illuminati. It is by no means exhaustive; there are many, many variations of specific techniques. I am also sure that different groups use different methods. If a survivor has memories that differ from what I have described, they must trust their own memories. I am only sharing what I remember about the Illuminati, a specific group I was a part of in Washington, DC and San Diego, California between

1957 and 1995.

My hope is that this article will help those who work with survivors or who wish to learn more about how these groups work. It will increase compassion for the enormous amount of suffering that a member of these groups undergoes and the struggle, once they leave, that they will have to overcome after those years of childhood conditioning. It takes remarkable courage to leave such a group, to say "no" to the pressure of the known, to decide to question values that have been accepted for years. To look at the suffering behind the programming and to cry for the manipulations and betrayals done since childhood.

TESTIMONY OF A SURVIVOR

Kim Campbell

Preliminary note from Svali: I wanted to publish a thought-provoking and courageous article written by a former Illuminatus who is still in recovery from the satanic ritual abuse he suffered. This article is being distributed with the permission of its author, Kim Campbell. My hope is that it will help educate Christians, and give hope to other victims of Satanism. The article itself was written in April 1999.

Testimony of my deliverance

My name is Kim Campbell. I'm 49 years old, and I live in Tulsa, Oklahoma. I'm married and happily so.

I work as a medical assistant and belong to Morning Star Testimony Church in Tulsa. Over the past few years, I have experienced the reality of my conversion to Christ through the personal choice I made.

In April 1993, I learned that I had a severe personality disorder due to the fact that I was born into a satanic family and had been subjected to satanic ritual abuse. I suffered from a split personality, which was dissociated into multiple personalities.

(**Translator's note**: This personality disorder is very common in those who have been ritually abused.

These traumas are designed to split their personality into a number of distinct personalities, each with its own identity and behavior. These different personalities, each with their own value systems, beliefs, emotions and experiences, can take turns taking control of the body in service of Satan's plan. These various personalities are not demons, although demons can control them. This splitting of the personality allows the victims of ritual abuse to better cope with the very violent traumas they have suffered, and to perform acts that their apparent "normal" personality would not allow them to do. Only the Lord can fully heal and restore these victims. See the page: http://www.pedopolis.com/pages/themes/mk-mind-kontrol-sous-pages/dossier-trouble-dissociatif-de-l-identite-anciennement-nomme-trouble-de-la-personnalite-multiple.html)

I must say that my deliverance from this satanic culture was the main trial of my life. The years I have been through have been difficult, but I believe my problems were largely resolved about three years ago. This profound crisis in my life marked the beginning of a genuine faith in Jesus Christ, the Savior and Lord of my life. I had always wanted to live such a faith, but I had never achieved it before.

This article is my testimony. I first wrote it in 1995. I hope that it will instruct those who minister to Illuminati survivors, especially the Shield of Faith Ministry in Minneapolis, which invited me to share my testimony. First and foremost, I want to give testimony of God's love for me, and for all members of the Body of His Son. I am absolutely amazed by this Father, Son and Holy Spirit God, who wants to show His divine glory, a glory that He delights to share with me, His son. With me, and with all His children! ! What a wonderful grace indeed!

My Satanic roots go back to both branches of my family. My "official" family are West Texas Texans, who taught me to tie my shoes, do my arithmetic homework, and be polite. These are normal things that most parents do for their children. Yet, a keen observer would have noticed the tendency toward depression, restlessness, and unbalanced behavior that characterized me. But, in a way, I was privileged. No one had diagnosed my severe personality disorder at that time. So I was apparently just another kid, albeit a very strange one.

However, behind this apparent veneer, I was also the direct descendant of a very ancient family immersed in an ancient satanic culture. This culture has secretly survived for thousands of years. It is as old as humanity. In this culture, people worship Satan as their god. Their worship of him, as well as their entire lifestyle, has always been imbued with a terrible violence.

By being part of this culture, I was exposed to all kinds of abuse, trauma and demonic influences that are typical of Satanism. This culture is incredibly evil, because it is controlled by the evil genie. Almost everything in this culture is designed to destroy human beings.

I reacted as all children react in this culture: by dissociating my personality.

All my life, from my earliest childhood, I have been subjected to traumas designed to develop my ability to fragment my personality. I have experienced all kinds of forced violence, both as a victim and as an executioner. I was put through very sophisticated mental programming programs here in the US, often in public clinics and institutions, as well as at the Tavistock Institute in England. I was indoctrinated into the Cabal, and was taken through all sorts of occult initiations, into the most ancient form of Satanism, the Sumerian-Akkadian mystery religion, the one practiced in Babylon.

So my personality was deliberately fragmented into separate elements, and all these multiple personalities were constructed and developed into my overall identity.

This culture is, of course, completely permeated by the power of demonic spirits. All these demons have become part of my life and even my nature. In a culture that is dedicated to the pursuit of power, demons are the ultimate resort. In American culture, people seek comfort, status and prestige. But in Satanic culture, people eagerly seek the power of demons.

Satanism has invaded all of Western civilization. Satanism is at the root of what we call today "paganism", in its ancient or contemporary forms. Satanism has developed over the millennia, gradually becoming part of the culture and power structures of all Western nations. It has its adherents in all areas of society, at all levels, and in all social strata. Satanism has had a profound influence on the intellectual life of the West over the past centuries. Its doctrines and writings have shaped Western thought, from the Greek philosophers, through St. Augustine, St. Thomas Aquinas, the Christian mystics of the 13th century, to the modern charismatic movement. Descartes, Spinoza, Kant, the philosophers of the Enlightenment, and many others, came from this satanic culture. Polynesian religion, animism, spiritualism, the religion of the American Indians, the Mayan and Inca cultures, the culture of ancient Egypt and Greece all stem from Satanism.

To believe that Satanic culture is all about ritual abuse is to demonstrate a fundamental ignorance of Satanism and its destructive influence in human history. Satanism has influenced politics, economics, art and music. To extend its influence, Satanism has always used the psycho-spiritual process called "personality disassociation". This practice of disassociation is as old as humanity itself.

This was the culture in which I was born and raised. The least I can say is that this culture is completely opposed to the Kingdom of God. These two cultures have never stopped fighting each other. And I can say that, since my birth, I have lived in the midst of this struggle. While I was a practicing Satanist, I also earned a Master's degree in Theology in 1976! I openly claimed to be a Christian, but my public life demonstrated the contradictions of living in two irreconcilable cultures. My love for the Lord was superficial. I deeply desired to love and be loved by Him, but I was unable to overcome my anxieties and doubts about the existence and character of God. My social life reflected an apparent relative success, but my spiritual life and relationships with others were a failure.

When I learned that I had this personality disorder caused by ritual abuse, I felt a deep emotional shock. But it was also the real starting point for me on the path to the Lord. For the first time in my life, I decided that the priority for me was to become the Christian I had always wanted to be. I knew that this was going to be very difficult, but I knew that if I was going to become a follower of Jesus Christ, I had to be completely free of the occult and healed of the fragmentation of my personality.

If I had to rely on the best methods and techniques of psychology and psychiatry, I knew I would never have had the money or the time. The traditional specialists could not have done anything for me. To this day, I am convinced that there is no traditional approach to dealing with a personality fragmented by Satanic ritual abuse. To be freed, I had no choice but to be freed by Jesus Christ.

For this reason, I took my relationship as a follower of Jesus Christ very seriously. Constantly, the Lord called me to holiness and spoke to me of the power of His love. He had forgiven me through His Son, and could deliver me from the power of sin. Every day after work, instead of "living normally," I stayed home to read, pray, cast out demons and claim my humanity. I would connect with my different split personalities, the ones that were accessible to me, to merge them and integrate them into the reality of my life. I learned all I could about personality dissociation, ritual abuse, and the healing process, in order to apply this knowledge to my own deliverance. I joined a church to hear from the Lord because my heavenly Father had chosen to use the "foolishness of the preaching of the cross" as the ultimate means of restructuring my personality. I attended prayer meetings where the presence and power of the Lord produced miracles in me and others. I scrutinized my life in the light of the Living Word of God. I submitted to the Lord's sanctifying work every sin committed by my various personalities, consciously or passively. After all, this fragmentation of my personality was none other than the sin par excellence. As a sinner,

I needed repentance and forgiveness above all. So I received my deliverance in obedience to the Lord.

When I found myself in a bind, or the obstacles were too difficult for me, I spent time with my pastor, Doug Riggs, who imparted the love and power of the Lord to me. Instead of spending hours getting my different personalities to talk, the Lord would allow us to go deep into the events that had shaped my personality. In fact, it consisted of vigorously casting out demons, and praying to our Father to allow me to merge my various personalities. My pastor also showed me, from the Bible, and in the light of the Person of Jesus Christ, how the abuse I had suffered had shaped my life. The Lord allowed me, through my pastor, to go much deeper than if I had been alone. He used him to convey His Word of grace to me, a man with a disassociated personality. Through the voice and presence of my pastor, the Lord made Himself more real to me. Many times, the Lord gave my pastor revelations and direction that were essential for me to solve the crises I was going through. The Lord uses men like him, and like so many others in the Body of Christ, to help men like me.

The Lord is not intimidated by darkness. After all, the good news is that he loved me while I was still in darkness. The Lord did all of this in the context of a small, seemingly insignificant local church of thirty or forty people (counting children), most of whom had undergone satanic ritual abuse or had a disassociated personality! We had banded together to work to hasten the Lord's return for His Bride, while in the occult our job was to fight against God's will for the Church, and to promote the coming of the Antichrist. As Christians, we prayed for each other, exhorted and counseled each other, while as Satanists we dominated and persecuted each other.

In "working out our salvation with fear and trembling," we were often compelled by the Living Word of God to remove the beams in our own eyes as we strove to remove the straws in the eyes of our brothers. The Lord was purifying us to teach us repentance. It was the Living Christ working in His Body, as He did in Capernaum before His crucifixion, or in Corinth after Pentecost.

This is how the Lord worked in my life as one of His disciples. Little by little, my Heavenly Father was delivering me, literally, from the moral and demonic power of sin, through the Person of His Son, the risen and living Jesus of Nazareth. Throughout this process, I never ceased to be amazed at the grace and power of God through His Son Jesus Christ.

After eighteen months of hard work, I still had multiple personalities. The Lord had told us to be bold. I had learned to recognize that the only real obstacle was myself. Not the hidden spiritual inner self, but the conscious outer self. Frankly, I was afraid to learn how bad I had been and perhaps still was. So the Lord made me realize that I had to face myself, and accept to be confronted with what I feared the most.

I was much worse than I thought!

In my mind, I thought of Satanic ritual abuse in the following way: these were extremely evil people who took nice little children and turned them into Satanists. I was wrong. We had been working for eighteen months to strip away the surface. But underneath, in the heart of my human personality, there was the nature of a Satanist! In truth, as far back as I could remember, I had been indoctrinated into a culture worthy of Sodom and Gomorrah, in a small brick house in West Texas. The Satanic abuse I had suffered did not change the fact that I was already living in a "normal" pagan culture! Everything I had experienced during those first eighteen months of deliverance work was really just a way to protect and hide the real nature of my true carnal self. I was now faced with the heart of the matter: I belonged to generations of Satanists. This was more than demonic possession. I was touching the deep reality of my human personality. It was the world I had lived in. I was the historical descendant of ancestors who had all practiced incest, violence and idolatry. As such, I was as demonized as the worst of the Canaanites!

But again, the Lord's grace was wonderful. Whatever was done, my God, my Heavenly Father, absolutely believes in the efficacy of the Sacrifice of His own Son on the Cross to wash away all our sin. In spite of the disgust and repulsion I felt for myself, this did not change the love and tenderness of the Lord for me. On the contrary, this tenderness and love became deeper, richer and more powerful. The Lord Jesus would not call my sin anything other than what it was. He would not allow me any excuses, nor would he tolerate any irresponsibility on my part. He did not need to diminish the seriousness of my sin, for His sacrifice was more than enough to erase it and give me new life.

So I learned that evil was not the greatest power in the universe. As God's grace and power freed my faculties to hear His voice and believe, I could better understand the nature of His relationship with me. It was only through this encouragement that I was able to continue to face the truth about my life and persevere on the path to deliverance.

So here is the structure of my personality as the Lord revealed it to me.

First, on the surface, there was a "good me" composed of my various personalities who worked, acted, went through marriage and divorce, and lived together in a "Christian" way. It was also this "me" that had to rediscover my entire deep past. Underneath this surface was what I will call a "dissociative layer". It was made up of the residual consequences of all the violence and demonic traumas I had suffered, and which were intended to reinforce my multiple dissociated personalities. It was this "layer" that gave great difficulty to the various therapists who had worked with me, who thought they were moving towards a solution, while the core of the problem remained hidden, undetected. At the deepest level, there was finally the hidden center of my human personality, the repository of all the abominable things practiced by my ancestors in the past generations. I had forgotten that this "hidden center" was completely opposite to the surface "good self" that I thought was my true personality.

Some say that people can be defined by what limits or shackles them, and I believe this is true. The core of my personality had been shaped by my emotional and affective attachment to the people who had played the most important role in my life. My original identity had been shaped by the emotional ties I had formed with those closest to me.

My mother's name was Lula Vieta Pauline Russel Campbell. She was born in 1917 in Farmersville, Texas and died in 1977. The man I knew as my father was not my real biological father. My real father, the man I loved and called "Dad," was Edouard Philippe de Rothschild. I was his natural son, named Philippe Eugène. This man was my father. As for me, I was the fruit of an occult incest, one of the hundreds of thousands of descendants, both legitimate and illegitimate, of this powerful financial and occult dynasty.

What was my life like in this family? For most of my childhood and teenage years, I lived with my father on his estate in France. I can remember how he spoke to me when I was a young boy. I remember his love of life and his passion for all things human. His god was humanity. He believed it with all his soul. He could talk for hours about the phenomenal achievements of the human race. He would take me to his library and spend long periods of time telling me about the miracles of mankind. I also loved the physical relationship we had. He was a firm believer in the emotional power of incest. In his culture, it was something "normal" and even worthy of admiration. I listened to him, and he passed on to me his intense taste for power, and even his hatred of God. This man enjoyed hating God, and I was his natural son. Such was the deep nature of the iniquity I had inherited from my ancestors.

Being a descendant of the Rothschilds, I could not have been more demonically inhabited!

How can it be that a child belonging to such a family can become a Christian? It must be known that the families of Satanists have this particularity, that they bring their own children into contact with the Gospel, in order to be able to destroy afterwards everything that makes the emotional power of a true faith. I remember how my father, on the advice of Dr. Joseph Mengele himself, led me to Christ. Dr. Joseph Mengele was the famous Nazi doctor who organized the elimination of Jews in the death camps and who directed the abominable "medical" experiments performed on the prisoners. He remained untraceable after the war).

His first clumsy attempts often failed, which earned him the harsh reproaches of the Doctor. But one day he succeeded. I understood the miracle by which God can become our Father. My heart opened ardently to this Holy God, who became my Father, my "Abba". Then my father and Dr. Mengele, through a perversion of the message of Scripture, led me to "put to death the old man" (our unregenerate human nature, according to the theology of the apostle Paul). They actually put me through a clinical death and "resurrected" me by medical means. I was just the tender age of two. Then they placed me in front of the "choice" of loving my Heavenly Father, who had led me to death, or my earthly father, who had brought me back to life. For a long time, my father reinforced these two contradictory desires in me: to belong to the Lord, or to belong to my earthly father. He worked to create in me an incredible internal tension between these two diametrically opposed emotional bonds. He did not allow me to resolve this tension on the level of my personality. This was the greatest struggle of my life, which led to an emotional and psychological disorder of the first magnitude. This conflict was later compounded by programmed abuse and carefully controlled conditioning of my personality using sophisticated medical techniques.

All this ends up producing a real split personality.

Thus, although I had truly become a Christian, after having felt the wonderful experience of the presence of the Holy Spirit within me, and after having received eternal life in Christ, I was immediately and deliberately deprived of these glorious realities, which were no longer available to me as a basis for my personality development. After truly experiencing my Christian identity, I was immediately indoctrinated back into the satanic culture. The ritual abuse that I subsequently suffered was to build a completely satanic edifice on this Christian foundation!

I was present when my father died in 1988. I received his power, and he entrusted me with the mission of pursuing my destiny in the great family conspiracy. Like the other children of the Rothschild dynasty, I played a vital role in my family's revolt against God. When I watch the news on television, I am amazed to see so many familiar faces taking center stage in all areas of politics, the arts, finance, fashion and business. I grew up with all of these people, and I would meet them in places where we practiced our satanic rituals, as well as in the "power centers."

Financiers, artists, royalty, and even Presidents and Heads of State, all were people with disassociated personalities, who are now working and conspiring to bring humanity into a New World Order, where the human being occupies the highest place, and God is only a faceless abstraction. All these people, like me, had undergone satanic ritual abuse that had dissociated their personality. Like the hundreds of thousands of other biological children in my occult family, I had my place and function in our family's plan to control the world. My efforts, as well as those of my family, were constantly directed toward recruiting a member of the European nobility of the Habsburg family to take the top position at the head of humanity, which is none other than the Antichrist of the Bible.

While other members of my family were assigned to infiltrate the government, universities, business and arts, my assigned place was within the Church, the Body of Christ. I was to be a center of spiritual power, and control satanic activity in the Church. All my life I had been in contact with people who were part of the Church, while channeling and spreading the satanic power of the False Prophet and Antichrist through the Rothschild family. From my childhood, I had been dedicated and trained in the vital task of carefully maintaining contact with the ancestral spiritual power of the False Prophet and Antichrist. All of us who were born into Satanist families, and who had been trained for decades to exert this influence in the Church, were all in contact within a local church. Our goal was to use the Church, the Body of Christ, as a means to manifest the False Prophet and Antichrist. Amazing!

There are many Christians in the Church with disassociated personalities who hold similar occult spiritual positions and who work for the satanic New World Order. I represented the "morning star" of

Lucifer, infiltrated into the Church. I was the representative of all the other Satanists who were in relationship with me, and who together constituted this "morning star". In the Church, their spirits were present in me.

So I was, in the Body of Christ, a mere human being, but also a spiritual center of collective Satanic energy. I had been trained in all sorts of rituals and was inhabited by powerful legions of evil spirits.

It was the Rothschilds in my family who trained me to occupy this occult spiritual position as a "morning star". This whole Satanic edifice was built on the foundation of my initial experience as a Christian! Outwardly, I was a false Christian, programmed to be hyper-pious, hypocritical and super spiritual.

But, as a Satanist belonging to the Rothschild family, I still had to go through a real experience of accepting Jesus Christ as my Lord at the tender age of two years and four months. That was the foundation of my personality.

However, it is precisely this experience that was crucial in my deliverance, as well as in my life as a Christian.

It was my conversion to Christ that was the fundamental event in my life. Afterwards, I was deliberately deprived of the benefits of this event and of my true identity. I was prevented from allowing my Christian faith to manifest itself in my behavior. I had lost the most important driving force of my personality.

I wonder if my deliverance would have been quicker if those who counseled me had first dealt with my biological and emotional identity as a Rothschild and my conversion to Christ as a child, with all the events that accompanied that conversion. For these were the initial factors that had caused the dissociation of my personality. If we had solved this basic problem, I believe that my disassociated personality would have been stripped of all the demonic, psychological and biological elements that had constituted it, and that this demonic system would have virtually collapsed.

My experience is far from unique. Everyone who has gone through a similar deliverance has gone through similar experiences. We all received Christ as children and then went through tremendous emotional conflict, torn between our attachment to God and our attachment to our parents. This conflict led to a fracture, a dissociation of our personality. This resulted in us being invaded by legions of evil spirits. It was the multiple personalities created as a result of this dissociation that were used by Satan. Subsequently, new personalities were created, forming a whole complex psychological system in the service of the Evil One.

For the Rothschilds, as I am sure it was for Satan himself, this was a perfect example of demonic irony and sadism. There is a form of Satanic genius in using Christians to work for the manifestation of the Antichrist! By infiltrating the entire Body of Christ, through its occult servants, Satan has been able to generate the spiritual and sociological forces required to establish the reign of the False Prophet and Antichrist. Such a conspiracy also prevents the Body of Christ from growing to the measure of the perfect stature of Christ, and from fully satisfying God's heart for His people. It is all these satanic infiltrations, both within and without the Body of Christ, that are the source of demonic energy, heresies, and all the actions that will result in the great apostasy foretold in 2 Thessalonians 2:3. It is then that the Antichrist, the son of perdition, will manifest himself.

Within all historical denominations, in the Ecumenical Movement, in the Word of Faith Movement, in parts of the Vineyard Movement, and especially in the charismatic heresies passed on within the "spiritual renewal" among Methodists and Presbyterians (among many others), in all the "occult Christian" practices of the movements seeking "church unity by signs, wonders and miracles", which were initiated by the heretical ministry of Oral Roberts, everywhere Satan has succeeded in seducing and worshipping himself as a god.

The visions and messages proclaimed by all these "ministries" are only the demonic projections of seducing spirits, which express themselves through the mouths of all these false prophets. Their miracles are only the acts produced by sorcerers who know neither the Father nor the Son. In Matthew 7, Jesus spoke about these false prophets, saying:

"Many will say to me on that day, 'Lord, Lord, have we not prophesied by your name? Have we not cast out demons by your name? And have we not done many miracles in your name? Then I will say to them openly: I never knew you; depart from me, you who do iniquity" (Matthew 7:22-23).

No matter how sincere the people who follow these movements may be, no matter how sublime, wonderful and ecstatic the experiences they may have, these movements are not from God. If the judgment begins with the house of God, there is good reason for it. Satan has used occult ritual abuse, and the phenomenon of personality disassociation, to infiltrate the Church with his false prophets, accompanied by their false spiritual gifts. The devil has practically succeeded in taking over the Church and holding it hostage to his interests, like a hijacker takes over an airliner.

Thus, not only are all areas of politics, social life and economics ready for the Antichrist, but also those of religion and spiritual life, including the visible Church of Christ.

The picture of a world headed for Hell, taking the Church with it, is a rather bleak and discouraging one. But the Bible is perfectly clear on this point: the period immediately preceding the return of Jesus Christ corresponds to this picture before our eyes. If you believe that the true church will be anything more than a weak faithful remnant in the midst of violence and deep darkness, you are sadly mistaken, and you do not know how to read the Scriptures.

The Lord God knows what He is doing. His omniscience, and the grace that flows from His Being, are more than enough for His true Church to persevere in faith and endure such evil power. My life is a living proof of this. What could my deliverance, and that of others like me, mean, if not that Jesus Christ is alive and working today? And that He has decided, in His sovereign grace, to bestow the incomprehensible riches of Christ on the paralyzed, the lame, the despised and the brokenhearted, to make us His covenant people, "that the principalities and powers in the heavenly places may know today through the church the manifold wisdom of God" (Ephesians 3:8-10).

Complete victory was not achieved by simply overcoming the demonic and disassociative bonds of this satanic conspiracy. I believe that the true joy our Father experienced in leading us to get rid of our problems and accomplish such a task was given to Him by the fact that He Himself gave us this moral victory over Satan and his evil powers through our relationship with our Heavenly Father and each other. This moral victory can be seen in the love we have for each other in our small assembly.

The obstacles are certainly formidable when it comes to being freed from our deeply demonic roots, and continuing to be faithful to the Lord in the midst of a world that is running toward Hell. But it is all worth it.

For our Father has brought us out of the swamp where we were sinking, to form disciples who, in their personal lives as well as in their mutual relationships, have given Satan a moral and spiritual defeat. In this struggle, both personal and collective, the Lord is fulfilling His desire: "that they may all be one, as you, Father, are in me, and I in you, that they also may be one in us, so that the world may believe that you have sent me. I have given them the glory that you have given me, that they may be one as we are one, I in them and you in me, that they may be perfectly one, and that the world may know that you sent me and loved them as you loved me" (John 17:21-23).

Because of my split personality, I had never been able to enter into a real Christian life, nor into God's will for me. By God's grace, I have now entered into it, and I have chosen to overcome the evil in me.

"He who overcomes will inherit these things; I will be his God, and he will be my son" (Rev. 21:7). Despite the manipulation and betrayal I had experienced, the decision to trust Jesus Christ, a decision I had made in my early childhood, was the right one. I am an ordinary person. As a Christian, I am not a superman. There are people in our little congregation, and in others, who have shown greater qualities of perseverance, courage, honesty and humility. There are many other Christians, with disassociated personalities or not, who, in responding to the call of Jesus to be His disciples, have been led to extraordinary depths of suffering and love for the Name of Jesus Christ. The world is not worthy of such Christians.

All my life the Lord has called me to trust and obey Him, as He calls every man to do.

How could I say to Him, "No!" The Son of God our Father, in His grace, "imprisoned" me and held me captive. It was because He claimed my life that I was able to keep a sense of reality enough to believe that He really existed, that I owed Him my life and love, and that His grace surpassed anything that had ever existed.

POLYFRAGMENTATION

Coping mechanism for the survivor

Note: the following article may seem like gibberish to someone who has never heard of dissociation and independent alters before... I imagine that for the author of the article (*Svali - 2000*), expressing in words these different possible personalities in a being is already complicated, the translation into French is just as complicated.

This subject of mental programming by fragmentation of a personality is surely one of the most complex to grasp. Some people will reject it out of hand, because it seems too far-fetched. For those who do, we invite them to first look at what is called Dissociative Identity Disorder in psychiatry, formerly called *"Multiple Personality"*. This is a starting point for understanding that a human can eventually be methodically programmed by undergoing repetitive traumas, creating independent personalities. If you wish to explore this further to determine whether it is fantasy or reality, you can consult these pages and give us your feedback:

Important Note: This article is not intended to be therapy nor is it a substitute for follow-up with a qualified and competent person, which is essential for healing from severe trauma. This article is only the opinion of a survivor. Trigger warning: content on ritual abuse, dissociation and trauma.

To survive ritual abuse, a child learns to disassociate, it disassociates strongly. The child suffers some of the most horrific abuse imaginable and most find a way to *protect* themselves. One of the ways that is encouraged in some groups is to create a complex defense system. In psychological terms, it is to fragment the child over and over again... Eventually the child becomes polyfragmented.

What is polyfragmentation? The term comes from the root "poly", which means "many" fragments. In complex polyfragmentation, the victim will have a system of alters, hundreds or even thousands of fragments. These are isolated pieces of their mind created to do a job efficiently and without thinking.

Often this work would be something abhorrent to the core personality. The further one is from the beliefs/morals of that core personality, the more dissociation/fragmentation must occur.

In other words, a person has to go through a lot of trauma to get them to do things they would never agree to do. And the person must feel very far from themselves when they do these things. The cult/cult will purposely create this polyfragmentation for this very reason, and it is also a way to facilitate control.

How are these polyfragmented systems structured?

These are individualities, they vary not only from person to person, but also in relation to the group to which the person belongs, in relation to the trainer, to the child's abilities and to the tasks that the child will have to accomplish. There is no standard recipe for creating polyfragmentation, but there are certain characteristics that are common.

What does a polyfragmented system look like?

I will share with you some of the basics of my memories when I was a trainer in this group myself, as well as some things about my own healing.

1 - Protective alters

These are fragments that were created to do the job that needs to be done, and save the life of the little child.

The protectors must look scary, just like the child's tormentors. They will also become tormentors when the child is an adult, because they have no choice. They can be ruthless, angry, or make it look like they are demons. Some growl, hiss, think they are powerful animals. At their core they were all a little child who was asked to do the unthinkable, who was forced to act in a way he or she didn't want to. They don't care about vulnerability and don't trust anyone, for good reason, their own experience in the cult. With therapy and time, they can also help the victim to get away from the abusers.

2 - Intellectual alters

The cult WANTS intellectual alters who can observe, go from one system to another, learn information quickly to send it out. This can be through recorders, computers, researchers. They can know several languages, master different philosophies. Brilliant and cognitive, they often think they can outwit those around them, including therapists. They know *the "story of life"* better than anyone else, as they rarely have strong feelings. These alters can *"read the life story"* without shedding a tear of emotion. When they are out, the person seems "flat", to say the least.

3 - The alters of denial

They are intellectuals and are created to deny that anything bad ever happened. Life was wonderful, perfect and loving parents and for these alters, suicidal tendencies and PTSD: http://www.pedopolis.com/blog/l-etat-de-stress-post-traumatique-espt.html are strange artifacts with no real reason to exist. A person can have a full-blown abreaction, and 5 minutes later, denial will come in to say it was all a fabrication. They are often frightened by the pain the person might have in remembering the severe trauma, that is what motivates them.

4 - The alternative controllers/"Head Honchos"/"Top Dogs

They are the leaders of the system, they know what is going on in the system at any given time. In a military system, it could be the general. In a protective system, the most powerful protector. In a metal system, the platinum. Or in a jewel system, the highest jewel like diamond, ruby or emerald.

Usually there are several leaders who share responsibility in a system. They can also become a valuable help over time if they choose to give up loyalty to the cult.

5 - Alternate children

They want praise from their adult leaders, who often give rewards or candy... They are also the "heart" of a polyfragmented system and can feel love, joy or terror. Often they want hugs and to be told they are "okay".

6 - The alters who punish

Why wait for an outside person to come and punish if you can create someone inside who can do it? Children will often identify strongly with their tormentors, and if the punishment is severe and frequent, they will internalize that tormentor to try to keep themselves "in line" and avoid punishment from outside. The sect will bank on this and often the programmer will leave as a *"visiting card"* an alter named by himself. This person will be an internal trainer, a "punisher" or an enforcer. Their job will be to try to keep things in line, and they will often try to sabotage the therapy. They are often afraid of external punishment if they do not do their job. The punishing alter will also activate sequences of self-punishment: programming for *"flooding,"* self-destruction, or suicide if the person begins to break with the cult and its rules. These fragments/alters may take time to be convinced that they can change these old ways, as they are held accountable to the programmer if things don't go their way.

7 - The alters of feelings

The feelings were overwhelming and endlessly traumatic during childhood. They threatened survival and sanity. The solution? Divide the feeling into internal parts/fragments. Divide the feeling in a way that is manageable. These alter feelings are often buried deep, and when they come out in therapy, it can be violent at first. A child's alter may come out screaming, in terror, or wailing in uncontrollable pain until brought back into the present moment. Often, feelings are heavily sanctioned in the cult, so it was psychologically necessary to bury them deep in the psyche in order to survive. These fragments can be very separate/remote from other alters who know what happened to cause such feelings, so they will seem to come out of nowhere, without any cause. With time and healing, they can connect with the intellectual alters who have observed this from the inside, and with others who have gone through the same trauma, making sense of the feelings and helping to resolve them.

8 - Internal advice

Most cults have councils and many members have internalized them, directly into themselves. This is another example of internalizing the tormentors, and these alters have a vested interest in keeping things in place/right, until they realize they can leave the cult/sect to be safe. Then they can become a tremendous force for healing. A person may have an internalized local governing council, or a spiritual council representing outsiders, such as an *internal* Druidic council or a group of *ascended masters* helping to make things work from within.

9 - Sexual alters

They are created to be able to deal with the traumas/violations that happened during early childhood when they reached sexual maturity.

They feel that it is too much for a small child to understand. Some have had to learn to *"enjoy"* the abuse, or pretend to enjoy it, and thus be highly rewarded for it.

10 - Amnesiac alters

These are called *"the clueless"*, *"those who know nothing"*, etc. They have the task of not remembering, otherwise, like a child, they are heavily punished. Usually they are very happy not to remember anything, and sometimes other alters who have been abused envy them or dislike their "protected" background. This can create hostility or war within the system until the amnesiac alters begin to accept that there was abuse. Reminding the abused alters that the amnesia saved the child (and their lives) and thus helped the system.

11 - Alter workers

They have jobs in everyday life and are usually part of the representative system (Public *Mode/Political Correctness*). They manage household chores, have married, take care of children, and may hold jobs with high responsibility. They are competent alters created to hide the fact that they have been subjected to traumatic violence and humiliation/degradation. These parts can be a great help to the other more traumatized and buried alters, as they show that life can be *"good"*.

12 - The other hosts

There may be a *"day host"* (see above), a *"night host"* (for worship), or hosts for various times in the person's life. Occasionally, the survivor may discover to his or her dismay that much of his or her life has been devoted to cult activities, or the night host is stronger than the day host. This is what happened to me. Fortunately, my night host is the one who left the cult, he had a lot of strength to pull us away from the group. I also had a host that was created during summers spent in Europe during my childhood. Also a *"hidden host"* who never fully showed up, this was to protect himself from the others (he manipulated the working alters to tell them what to do). Each system will handle this task differently. In general, the more severe the trauma, the more distrust there will be from outsiders and the more the host will have a façade, a strong protection.

13 - The basic core

This is the original child, the one who created all the others inside. The child's system will depend on the trauma and creativity of the original child, as well as its need to protect itself from the abuse of others that might have destroyed it. In some systems, the core is very young, if the abuse and severity began at an extremely early age. These cores often involve the parents or parental figures who caused the severe trauma. This includes forms of abandonment, torture and other cruelty to the young child.

14 - The divided core

This can be done again through severe trauma in early childhood. This is usually practiced by some groups to create larger, even more dissociated systems. (fragmentation of personality fragments...)

15 - Function codes, access codes

These are fragments created to perform certain tasks, they are created to do a job only when called by a trigger, such as letters, numbers, phrases or other sound stimuli. These are created with deep trauma.

16 - The spiritual alters

These alters may have a variety of beliefs covering different spiritualities. There may be one dominant spiritual belief in the system, or even several. For example, a spiritual system created by the cult may include aspects of Luciferianism, Druidism, Set Temple teachings, Babylonian mystery religions, etc. A "host" or "worker" alter may have a totally contradictory belief system and there may be hostilities between alters with opposing beliefs. In my own life, my "hosts" (working alters, public figure) were devout Christians, which provided stability for healing buried alters. It also opened the way for forgiveness, one of the most difficult and important tasks in this healing process.

This was an overview of some of the personality types that can be found in a polyfragmented system. It is important to understand that each person is unique, that people deal with trauma in their own way. This is not to say that every survivor of these cults has all of these personalities/alters in them... My hope is that this article will help educate others on this topic and issue.

INTERVIEW WITH BRICE TAYLOR

B rice Taylor is a survivor of an MK-ULTRA program where she exposed the ritual abuse. She is the author of the book "Thanks for the memories: the truth has set me free", in which she exposes government intrigue and the use of "sex slaves" by people in high places. She is also the owner of EEG Spectrum, a brainwave therapy center in North Carolina. She kindly agreed to be interviewed for this article and share her feelings on this topic. It's worth listening to her, she is a courageous person and her fight for herself and her daughter is most inspiring.

Question: Brice, how did you come to speak out against ritual abuse and/or mind control? What motivated your decision? How did you find the courage to speak out?

Answer: I started speaking out about ritual abuse because I was in the process of healing from my past as a victim and my recovery seemed to require it. As a mother of three, I felt compelled to speak out to alert the public to what was happening and to help others who were suffering the same abuse. I never took the safe route. My life always felt like it was in danger, so I continued to speak out to keep myself safe and to provide help to my children and others. I don't know if I acted with what is called "courage" in making those whistleblowers, but my maternal instincts were and are so deep that I only did what I had to do - and that required me to do things that most people would find scary. Like being willing to risk my life by saying things publicly. Doing nothing was far more terrible to me, because I knew that this abuse would continue over and over again unless it was exposed and stopped. Love for my children and humanity remains my only driving force. And God remains my strength.

Question: How did you begin to recover your own trauma memories? What were the triggers for these memories? Did you seek to confirm your memories? If so, what did you find?

Answer: In the early 1980's I think I began to remember "unconsciously", but at that time it was always difficult for me to bring memories to my conscious mind because of the mind control program that was dictating my life at that time. The first attempts of my conscious mind to disclose the activities I was involved in resulted in migraines related to the programming. As soon as my unconscious experiences created a threat of disclosure of well locked secrets for national security reasons. I had an accident, a head-on collision, with my head hitting the windshield of the car. Although not severely injured on the surface, it seems that this blow to the forehead caused my two cerebral hemispheres to begin communicating in a new way. Memories began to flood into my consciousness, followed closely by programmed commands that made me think I was crazy, gave me migraines, caused me to call my controllers and report what I remembered, and/or made me want to kill myself.

At first I had to face my parents. It was difficult, but the truth was told. My mother cried when I told her my memories. I told her that she and the rest of the family were all part of the abuse I remembered. She never denied my memories, she said that she believed me, but that she herself had forgotten. She has been with me all these years and since she funded my first two books and advised me to tell the truth whatever it is, I think she believes it is all true, despite her lack of memories. Her tears spoke volumes. She actually wrote a chapter in my last book, which explains what she went through with the multiple personality disorder my father has and all the abuse the family went through. I am grateful for my mother's help in this, because what she wrote was a great help to other survivors and their families.

My recollections were confirmed in part by known sources. My recollections in government were further confirmed to me personally when I was approached by Secret Service agents. On one occasion, a White House Secret Service agent found himself (mysteriously!?) sitting next to me on an airplane and told me not to give names I would remember or talk. I didn't give names for many years when testifying in churches or meeting with mental health specialists. One of my biggest confirmations was to comply with the wishes of the White House Secret Service agent and not name names.

Often after my interviews (where I did not name the perpetrators), survivors and therapists would meet with me to have me name (in private) the people who had abused me. There were all kinds of threats during those years, too many to mention, but one that let me know that I was absolutely on the right track was when my office burned down, where my Spectrum equipment was located that I used to practice the latest stage of brainwave training with survivors. I guess this technology that helps trauma survivors learn how to stay alert and attentive and not dissociate is effective, shows that they didn't really want to see this opportunity for healing and release in service to others. To make sure I understood that this was not an accident, but a warning to cease and desist, they had placed two bags of ash from the fire in front of my house, which I could see from the kitchen window. Instead of giving up, I ordered three more EEG machines and was able to open an eight-room office, where I could receive more people for the beneficial effects of this brainwave training!

As survivors, we almost have to play it smart to get through the backlash in one piece, and certainly since the torture and torture conditioning, we are more used to the hard knocks than most people. We can take the hits if we want to. I choose this solution. I would never have survived otherwise. But that was then. Today it seems easier to get out of the organized groups of manipulators who try to control others because there are more and more professionals exposing ritual abuse and mind control, and survivors healing. We survivors are stepping into an important role - a role that cannot be ignored. I think the truth is emerging as never before and it's a very interesting time. I could never have imagined years ago that in the year 2000 I would be given the opportunity to reach millions of people on Channel 13 News to talk about ritual abuse and mind control and have my speech validated by a retired FBI chief and a therapist who spoke about the 60 survivors she has helped who say the same things I do! The FMSF psychiatrist

(False Memory Syndrome Foundation) interviewed, when asked outright if he was part of the CIA replied, "I don't know if I'm part of the CIA, maybe they do." What kind of answer is that?

Many, many survivors are being helped more and more to heal and their healing has paved the way for the great revelation of the facts to be revealed to the public. I think the experiences of survivors, put together, clearly identify the many issues that need to be brought to the forefront to be resolved. More and more people are listening and the truth is coming out in ways that I honestly never thought possible in my lifetime. I am encouraged by this.

SURVIVING TORTURE

I was four years old and tied to a chair. Padded straps immobilized my arms, wrists and feet, and my neck and head were trapped in a system that prevented any movement. A woman came up to me, speaking to me in a harsh German voice. When I didn't answer correctly, she approached me, her angry face right above my terrified one. Slowly, methodically, she would take the cigarette stuck between her lips and point it at my bare thigh. She kept the cigarette there while I screamed. The woman was my mother and the little round scar is still there today.

This is one of the most difficult topics for me to write about, but any discussion of ritual abuse is incomplete without addressing it. It's not a very popular topic, one that many would prefer to avoid. A topic that is quickly glossed over in discussions of ritual abuse by talking about "dysfunction," "trauma," "suffering" or "abuse." But for a child growing up in a satanic or luciferian cult, there is only one word that describes the reality experienced. That word is torture.

In these groups, children are subjected to physical, psychological and sexual torture in its most extreme form and must learn to cope with this overwhelming reality. They must live with the realization that the people torturing them are their parents, grandparents, aunts, uncles, cousins, and siblings and deal with the consequences of shame and betrayal. This article provides a view of the effects of torture through the eyes of the person who experiences it.

The Canadian Centre for Victims of Torture (CCVT) has a list of psychological symptoms that occur as a result of torture, in bulk: "anxiety, depression, irritability, paranoia, guilt, distrust, sexual dysfunction, loss of concentration, confusion, insomnia, nightmares, memory deficit and loss."

"These symptoms appear when an individual angrily rebels against the violation of his or her rightful territory, whether physical or psychological." The nightmares represent an unconscious search to resolve the awful pain of this trauma; the distrust and paranoia speak to the instinctive trust in humanity that has been irrevocably ruined. The person who has endured and survived the torture will never be the same again. Memory loss occurs when the psyche desperately tries to block out the horrors endured, often through dissociation or other blocking mechanism. The author continues:

"Survivors of torture are often reluctant to share information about their experiences. They may be suspicious, frightened, or try to forget what happened. Their feelings may discourage them from seeking the help they need."

This article was written for medical personnel dealing with victims of torture under totalitarian regimes in South America and other countries, but the symptoms are the same for the survivor of ritual abuse.

The individual often blames himself or herself for his or her past torture, especially if it happened in early childhood. Torture engraves within the individual a deep sense that something is wrong, something that causes others to abuse him or her. Nurses are advised, "For example, it is important to remember that those who seek psychiatric help are initially healthy people who have been systematically subjected to treatment designed to destroy their personality, sense of identity, confidence and ability to function in society..."

Survivors of ritual abuse often struggle with these same things. They are often clear, competent, high-functioning people who would be called gifted, but the destruction of their self has done so much damage that they will rarely be able to reach their social or emotional potential. Survivors of torture may fear medical procedures:

"Doctors (sometimes crossed paths in prison who come to learn about the amount of abuse torturers can put their victims through or how to cause maximum suffering without killing the victim)..."

Ritualistic doctors perform this same function, and will also use their medical skills to repair the damage done after a particularly intense session.

"Therapists need to understand that surgical and examination instruments and medical procedures may be the same as those used to torture, so all procedures should be carefully explained. Some treatments, such as physical therapy, need to be done with particular awareness of the possibility of a very limited threshold of suffering."

"Survivors of torture and their families may also lose some of the values and beliefs they held before they experienced the trauma. They may be unable to trust and become disillusioned as a result."

One of the common struggles that survivors of ritual abuse and torture report is a difficulty in the area of trust and intimacy. Even for those who escape ritual abuse, the constant fear of being taken away or returned to their torturers will instill a distrust of others. Only those who over time prove to be safe and reliable will be among the often very small circle of those the survivor trusts.

"Dr. Philip Berger, one of the founders of CCVT, explained that when he started his sessions on torture for medical professionals in 1977, he was not believed. He was told that torture probably existed somewhere and was sometimes practiced, but not to the extent that it required a specialized response. This denial works on several levels. Torture is a barbaric practice, which most people prefer to avoid. This denial operates on at least three levels: denial on the part of the victim; denial on the part of the helper; and denial on the part of society as a whole. It is the extent of this denial that authorizes both the practice of torture and the continuation and survival of its effects.

If this is true for documented torture of victims of totalitarian regimes around the world, how convincing is the defiance and denial for the continued torture of innocent children by occult groups! Society often practices total denial of this subject, or even denial of it, because to acknowledge it would mean losing the "comfort zone" where almost everyone lives. The challenge of healing for an individual who has endured a lifetime of torture is this: acknowledging feelings, including rage, experienced by acknowledging the powerlessness that resulted in a struggle against the deep inner resistance to remember or acknowledge what happened (it is not necessary to remember all the memories, but some acknowledgement of what happened is an important part of healing and integration). Learning that the survivor has the tools to change. Learning that it was NOT the survivor's fault (survivors will often carry around a low self-image in response to the torture). Learning to undo the messages given under torture, and replace them with real teaching to overcome the fear induced by the torture, to face an old belief system and old ways of acting. Realize that it was not God's fault (many survivors struggle with this idea, wondering why He allowed the torture, or why it was THEY who had to endure it). Forgiving those who tormented the survivor (only after going through the above steps).

Recognize the past and then look forward to a better today.

Torture often leaves lasting marks, both physical and psychological on the survivor, but with time and support, it is possible to heal. One aspect of healing is becoming aware of the lasting effects of torture, which is only now beginning to be documented in the medical literature, recognizing these symptoms if they occur, and taking steps toward relief and healing from the underlying causes.

Another aspect of healing will come when survivors of this extreme form of abuse are able to talk about it and when society stops denying what is happening and begins to act to stop the abuse.

INTERVIEW WITH JEANNIE RISEMAN

Occasionally there are survivors with a special gift who choose to use this ability to help other survivors. Jeannie Riseman is one such person. She is a talented writer and editor and the fruits of her labor can be seen in Survivorship magazine. Survivorship.org created by Caryn Stardancer, which Jeannie now edits.

Jeannie also created the home page for ritualabuse.us, one of the longest running (and one of the best!) resource sites on the web, whether you are a survivor who wants to testify about ritual abuse or a resource person or therapist who wants to find more information. She has spent hours gathering information and organizing it by index on her site.

Jeannie has graciously agreed to be interviewed and to share elements of her past with us.

Question: Jeannie, how did you come to speak out against ritual abuse and/or mind control? What made you make this decision? How did you find the courage to speak out?

Answer: It was instinctive. When I remembered my very first abuse, one of my first thoughts was "he's a politician." I started talking about it to everyone under the sun and haven't stopped talking since.

Q: How did you begin to remember your own trauma? Were there any triggers for this remembering process? Did you seek to validate your memories? If so, what did you find?

A: My parents and husband were deceased and my children were raised and on their own. I was only responsible for myself, which I thought was really key.

I'm actually one of the few people I know who found out about the abuse in therapy. My therapist, who I trusted and loved, decided to try a little Gestalt exercise where two people push each other away with their hands (which is supposed to make it easier to say "no" or something like that). Since he was very tall, he knelt down to get to my level and I saw myself in a flash at age 4 with a man on his knees doing his thing. My poor therapist didn't understand why I was sobbing and staying silent!

This released a host of memories, my first rape by a man, then memories of the group and the experience in the cult. I can't validate any of the memories, maybe because the generation before me are mostly dead. And ours was an oral tradition; we didn't keep anything in writing.

Q: What have been your experiences with either or both combinations for: a) cult control and programming b) government mind control c) any other kind of intentional abuse?

A: About five years ago, I was able to reconstruct an elaborate programming system, which I then wrote down. I gradually came to believe that I was one of the original New York mind control test subjects (in the 1940s). In my early teens, I was fired before I received the full programming. I think that project, or sub-project, was abandoned. I have never met anyone with programming like mine.

I don't know the names of the people involved or where it took place, but I think the people and the site(s) had to do with academia.

Q: Do you think there are organized groups that are engaged in this? Why do you think they are doing this to people?

A: Yes, without a doubt. They do it for power, either for personal advancement or for "national security.

Q: Many survivors struggle for treatment with a society that doesn't believe them, with their own inner pain, and the lack of validation from family members. What would you say to them? What do you think about these issues?

A: I have made the choice to surround myself with people who believe me, at least most of the time. I don't hang out with people who doubt me - I just say "well, I think we disagree" and let it go. There is a certain power in telling someone who may think if they feel like it that you are psychotic, that you don't care, and then acting completely sane and rational. I'm lucky that all the people I really love believe me.

Finally, Jeannie shares some great ideas on how survivors can support each other and the pitfalls to avoid:

It is important to communicate our experiences as much as possible - both about abuse and about healing. The more we know, the more we can put our experiences into context, the better. Communication touches the very foundation of programming by demonstrating that it is possible to talk and live to talk again. It counteracts isolation, feelings of being "crazy" and the lie that we "belong" to them forever.

I think it is important to avoid the gaze of others if we want to eliminate our suffering or "fix" ourselves, and it is also important not to try to control other survivors. None of us has all the answers: only collectively can we build a knowledge base about how to live with dignity after such extreme abuse.

HOW TO HELP A SURVIVOR

One of the most common questions I am asked is, "How can I help a survivor?" It is asked by wives, friends, church members, and represents the desire to want to be of some help. Hidden behind this question is often the veiled request, "I don't want to do anything harmful by mistake."

There is no magic formula or set of actions that guarantee this help. Each person is unique and he or she has different needs. I, for example, am NOT an expert in assistance. At the same time, I know that in my own personal healing endeavors and those with whom I have spoken, some things have been helpful, while for others it has been the opposite. This should only be an informal helping discussion and not therapeutic advice.

Okay, so what will be helpful to someone who is a survivor of ritual abuse, who is just beginning to remember, or who has been recovering memories for several years, or who is in the process of trying to leave a destructive cult group? Here are some ideas.

1) Listening. The survivor who has been harmed in a cult group has heard all his or her life that he or she should not talk about the abuse, that he or she should not say anything. This is called "the code of silence. Once the survivor begins to remember, he or she will still need to share with someone he or she trusts. Ideally, this person will be his or her therapist, but he or she may want to share with a friend his or her feelings, his or her doubts, his or her feelings of horror, his or her despair, and his or her joy at the small steps of healing and liberation that are beginning to occur. Above all, what is important is that the person listening BE PRESENT and not reject it. But be aware that what she is revealing may panic her or reset programming. So don't rush the person. Let them go at a pace they are comfortable with.

2) Believe. Survivors of occult groups have been told that no one will believe them if they talk (and for good reason: much of today's society is in denial about this type of abuse!). The leaders of the group told him that they would be labeled as "crazy" and sent to a hospital, or branded as liars. This, along with the threat of severe punishment if they talk, makes many survivors reluctant to remember and tell about their abuse. If a survivor takes this important step, it is important to ratify it, even if what they reveal horrifies you or tests your own belief about human nature. What happened seems unbearable and the cruelty beyond human capacity, but often these initial facts are just the tip of the iceberg. Try never to tell the person that you don't believe them, otherwise you can say, in case they ask if you believe them, "I know you do and it doesn't matter what I personally think" (they will ask again and again because of the above mentioned programming that they will not be believed. Every time you say "yes" you are helping her break the power of the vicious cycle.

3) Learn about ritual abuse. It is one thing for you to listen to someone's story that tests your ability to believe them. But reading what thousands of people have written who remember these things will play on your gullibility and you will be able to educate yourself. Also learning a little more about ritual abuse will help you to know the possible pitfalls and problems the survivor faces during their journey. The best source of information is a caring therapist who knows about ritual abuse. If you want to contact one, let them know you are a resource and ask if you can meet with them and ask some questions.

Other sources may come from websites (like this one!). But don't go to just one; search multiple sites, as different survivors will have different perspectives.

At the library near you, there are at least a few books on the subject. (**note:** In France, you can always look for a book on multiple personalities/IDTs in a library, which would be a good starting point for the subject, but as for a French book on ritual abuse/mental programming...) Reading the story of a survivor and how he or she recovered can be helpful.

Conferences on ritual abuse can be excellent sources of information. You can contact national groups that deal with dissociation and attend their conferences.

4) Learn about programming. Many survivors of severe cult abuse will have experienced various forms of programming. You do not need to be an expert in programming to be supportive. But it is important to be aware that programming for self-harm and suicide, as well as the desire to reconnect with the cult (contact programming), can occur. If your friend states that he or she feels capable of self-harm, suicide or going to a cult meeting and feels that he or she cannot control his or her impulses, you should immediately put him or her in touch with his or her therapist. Hospitalization may be necessary if this urge is severe and a safe place to reduce programming. The therapist can also work with him as an outpatient to break the hold of the programming.

If the person reconnects with the cult, letting them know that they can live a good life outside the cult is important to escape the programming. That going back in will only get them deeper and that they can change their bad habits.

5) Having a good time, having fun, feeling safe, sharing distractions, such as going to a barbecue, shopping, thinking about crafts for fun are all things that can help a survivor who has been trapped in an emotionally deprived life (which makes him/her dependent on the cult). By discovering a different reality without abuse for the FIRST time in his life, childish sides may resurface. Give him the opportunity to express them and be aware that he may act in a way that is not related to his real age, i.e. easily infantile. The more healthy, appropriate experiences he has, the faster the healing will be, because his infantilism prevents the survivor from manifesting his emotional capacities. He will hurry to share this recourse and soon other elements will come out to "verify what is going on". In reality he will test the reliability of the friend and whether it is really possible to have a friend who does not abuse him and try to use him.

6) Lending a hand when things go wrong: Occasionally the survivor may experience chaotic moments, or have done a lot of inner work that otherwise leaves little room for much.

A close friend can help by taking him to therapy on those days if he can't drive. Small things can make a difference, like taking him in on a difficult day and cooking for him. Or just going out together and assuming the role of a safe outsider can often be enough.

7) Establish good marks: It is important not to do for the survivor what they can do for themselves. The idea is NOT to play the role of a parent, otherwise an unhealthy dynamic is created in the relationship. The survivor would have strong unmet dependency needs stemming from their emotionally deprived life. Let him/her know that you are his/her FRIEND. But not a nanny. There is a balance between helping out once in a while on really bad days and being overly dependent. Many survivors can function very well with everyday tasks, at least most of the time. Encourage them to do so. If the child side is constantly expressing itself, with no adult side showing, it may be a sign of stress in an overloaded system, a sign that it needs it (the adult sides were abused or punished and destroyed themselves), or a sign of unhealthy dependency. It is the survivor himself or herself who will learn to support himself or herself and a caring friend will encourage this.

8) Praying for him: I left for last what I think is most important. Healing from ritual abuse and leaving an occult group is the most intense spiritual battle of its kind. Any resource person can suffer a spiritual attack (and in rare cases physical threats as well). An unwavering faith, a knowledge of the means of spiritual warfare for you and your friend is the greatest gift of all. If they are open to Christianity, sharing their love and God's love can go a long way to nullifying the false beliefs about Him taught by the cult to the survivor. They will often show anger, rage, bitterness and even hatred for God and Jesus. Don't be shocked by this or walk away from the survivor for a while because he or she has suffered a lifetime of abuse and set up with God who was a rapist (it is hard to love Jesus when someone dressed like him raped you when you were a little child and you were told that this is what Jesus does to children).

With love, prayers and patience, this anger will subside and true healing of the survivor's greatest space of suffering, the spiritual, will begin. A survivor needs to see God's love in action in others, to see that the cult has lied to them, that Christianity is real, not just hypocrisy, and that Christians keep their word through prayer and acts of charity.

MK-ULTRA

PROGRAMMING AN ASSASSIN

In the coming months, I plan to write articles on Illuminati methods for more complex forms of programming. This one is the first in the series and I hope its information will be useful.

Since it is impossible to discuss programming without mentioning how it is done, please be aware, as a survivor of this type of abuse, that this reading may be a trigger.

Please protect yourself and read only when you are with your therapist or in a safe place.

One of the cruelest forms of training a young child has to undergo is to become an assassin, or to be able to take the life of another human being in cold blood on command. In the Illuminati group to which I belonged, almost every child and teenager had to undergo this military training.

The results are dramatic. The child must dissociate strongly to endure the ordeal of programming and the impossible demands on his psyche. A child can be taught and trained to do this, but he or she can never learn to be comfortable with the guilt involved.

Training often begins at a very young age. A two-year-old child is put in a metal cage connected to electrodes or is tortured on a table or chair. After a long time, he is released. He will feel dazed and will barely be able to walk. He is given a small animal, often a kitten, and told to wring its neck. The child will refuse. He will then be put back in the cage or electrodes will be attached again and he will receive another shock as punishment. He will be released again and told to wring the neck of a young animal. The child will cry and fear another torture. Trembling, he will finally do what he was ordered to do. Afterwards, he will often go into a corner to vomit, praised all the while by his trainer for the "good job" he did. The child will have created a fragmentation that obeys the trainer, to avoid the horrible suffering of disobedience (the greater the programming, the farther away it is from the child's basic natural values, the more severe the level of suffering used to create the programming). This is the first of a horrible series of steps. This continues over the years and the animals will get bigger and bigger. This is to desensitize the child to the concept of taking a life. During military training, the older children (between 7 and 10 years old) will learn how to handle a rifle with precision. They learn how to clean a gun, reload, unload, and shoot targets. They are highly rewarded for accuracy and reprimanded and punished if they make mistakes. By the age of twelve, most children do very well with a small pistol or rifle. They are then taken to a compound and taught to shoot animals that have been drugged to slow their movements slightly. The child learns to aim for the head or heart. The targets then turn into pictures of realistic human models.

And all the while, they are increasing their level of anger with the continued torture and abuse. The child is told to "use their anger" to increase their performance. During the virtual reality exercises, the animal targets are replaced by human targets. The child will learn to hit the "bad guys" and direct his or her rage at them. Accuracy in these exercises is rewarded and praised and mistakes are punished.

The child learns to obey a command code to start the "find the target" sequence and then to execute the "kill" sequence, which involves killing the target. Under drugs and hypnosis, the young teenager will be convinced that this is reality. One day he will be tested and told (in virtual reality, but he does not realize it under hypnosis) to shoot his parents or siblings, who are graphically simulated in the virtual reality program. Which they do.

At this point, the child is considered "reliable" on "command. If he or she shoots the person he or she loves the most on command, the programming is considered "ingrained," and now only needs to be reinforced periodically.

This sounds horrible, but this is how they trained an assassin in the group I was in.

I suffered it and had to put others through it. I regret it so much today. It was a perfectly planned process, with a step-by-step progression. No one gives a teenager a gun and says, "Go kill someone" in these groups, because the child would refuse and be unable to. They start at a pre-verbal age and develop each skill so that it overlaps with the others.

They rely on the young child's helplessness and rage towards others to fuel the programming.

Many of these techniques are based on MK ULTRA research done by the CIA in the 1960s and 1970s. The Illuminati trainers were in close contact with members of the military intelligence community who worked on these projects, such as Col. Aquinos, Sidney Gottlieb and Alan Dulles, among others. This knowledge of how to condition a subject was passed on to the trainers of the different groups and was put into practice with modifications according to age.

Children in the Illuminati are expected to complete such tasks in stages and advance to the next level as soon as they can demonstrate their mastery. An army commander will ask a young teenage leader to kill someone in front of the others with his bare hands to demonstrate his loyalty and obedience.

The teen will receive higher status and rewards for doing well and quickly.

This type of programming can be dismantled, with time, therapy and concerted effort, and especially prayer, to dissolve the horrible traumas that have been induced. No human being should be forced to do these things or undergo this form of training. It generates massive dissociation and intense grief when the person realizes what they have done. It helped me realize that:

- I had no choice at the time. As a young child, I was forced into it by older children. The alters created that learned to accept or even enjoy this training were put in place by the need for dissociation and psychological escape caused by this horrible trauma and these elements contain deep pain and injury.

- I can lay my burden at God's feet and lay my suffering and the lifelong wounds of intense pain and guilt that these experiences have caused others and know His forgiveness

- I now have a choice and I have chosen to move away from this type of activity

- I can pray that others will get away with this horrible kind of abuse

- I can express to God the anger and sense of outrage that this deliberate manipulation has brought upon myself and others, and find healing. This rage has often made it possible to endure past abuse and as diminishes, the hold of the programming can weaken as well.

This type of programming is the most insidious form of mind control and healing is possible. It is a long and slow process, but it is worth the effort.

EXPERIENCES ON THE EDGE OF DEATH

Programming by NDE

(**Note**: the content of this article discusses traumatic programming in detail and could be an important trigger for survivors who have experienced this type of abuse. If you are a survivor, please do not read unless you are with a reassuring person or your therapist) This article is part of an ongoing series I am writing as a draft on complex programming for the sequel to my first book, "Breaking the Chains". I'm going to talk about one of the most traumatic forms of programming a survivor can experience. This programming involves the use of near-death experiences. The Illuminati have been studying human neurophysiology and the effects of traumatic conditioning on the brain and psyche for years. In seeking better and more reliable methods of instilling programming, they have used research from a variety of sources: government agencies, totalitarian regimes, and their own ongoing (and secret) experiments.

But some of the fundamentals of this type of programming have been around for centuries. One of the oldest rituals used by the Illuminati is the "resurrection ceremony". The phoenix, a symbol of death and new life, is actually one of their most prized symbols, symbolizing the coming of the New Order and its leader.

How does resurrection programming or its variants work? I will share what I have experienced and/or witnessed.

A young child of about two or three years of age will be severely traumatized during an occult ceremony. He will be raped, beaten, electrocuted and even asphyxiated and given drugs that will create a near death state. The child will always feel presences hanging over his or her body at this time, watching the unconscious body that has been tortured to the point of near death. Competent medical personnel will always be involved in the programming of this death, monitoring the child's physical condition in order to resuscitate him or her.

They have resurrection equipment and medication on hand at all times. The child who has reached this point will cry in his heart and will regain consciousness in extreme pain. He will then be told that he has a "choice": face certain death or choose to live by inviting a powerful demon into him.

The child chooses life. A demon enters, the child sinks into unconsciousness and then awakens in clean clothes, in a soft bed, coated with healing ointments. He is extremely weak and shaken, and a gentle, caring female (or male) voice tells him that he is dead, but that the demon "brought him back to life," that he is indebted to it and to those who "saved" him from his life and heartbeat. The child is also told that if he asks the demonic entity to leave, he will be returned to the near-death state he was in when it entered.

This is one type of NDE experience used to control and terrify a very young child and to force him or her to accept a demonic spirituality under the most traumatic and coercive circumstances imaginable.

The child feels marked and chosen for life by this experience and it profoundly influences the child's own inner beliefs and most basic reality. It is also one of the most horrific manipulations a young child must undergo and is designed to take away their free will or choice.

Another form of borderline programming will occur under the conditions that have often been called "government mind control," but which I have always seen linked to Illuminati programming (as trainers/scientists on both sides have exchanged and shared information).

For example, at the Tulane Medical Center, there was a place called "The Institute" next door. The Institute was in the business of experimenting with mind control techniques performed under the most extreme circumstances, including at one point near physical death. For some of these programs, the "subject" (as I hate this word used by the trainers to distance themselves emotionally from the fact that he or she is a human being with feelings and emotions that are being worked on) goes to a room in the hospital isolated from the others by bare light gray walls. The subject is tied in four places and also at the waist and neck. He is then wrapped in a kind of cocoon of soft bandages that limits the movements or suppresses any sensation in the limbs.

The "subjects" are usually fed intravenously and then undergo severe sensory deprivation, bombarded by extremely loud noises. The darkness of the room will be interspersed with dazzling white lights in the middle of the night, and the "subject" will lose the sense of day and night.

The subject, almost broken, is then electro-shocked strongly and drugged. They may be put on a ventilator and given paralyzing drugs. The level of anxiety reaches extreme points as the abuse progresses and I have heard of people literally having heart attacks because of the fear experienced at that time. The person is drugged and shocked again and is told that they are dying. She sees her body from above and is actually happy at that point to finally be free of her days of torture.

Then a soft-spoken trainer comes along and says over and over again, "You deserve to live, I won't let you die. You owe me your life." Recorded messages are also played continuously that describe the future destiny of the "subjects" towards the "family", etc. Finally, slowly, the subject is allowed to wake up, to come out of his unconsciousness, accompanied by the constant message that he is "reborn" for the family group. Friendly faces comfort the subject as he or she recovers from this horribly traumatic programming sequence. The person feels extremely grateful to be alive, to be free of the horrors of those days when they lay in the Institute in a near death state and will clutch like a small child at the adults around them. She is very vulnerable at this time and extremely receptive to the messages embedded in trauma. I should know. I was a "subject" of the Institute as a child in the 60's and early 70's and then as an adult, as a "consultant".

This is intense level programming performed under extreme circumstances and the fear level of a survivor who begins to remember this type of trauma can be extremely high. I wish I could embellish, say it's not so bad, but it really is. I know some people will be incredulous, but this type of programming really does exist (along with other types of sophisticated mind control methods). There are many variations of death-border programming, and I'm only touching on two of them (there are other forms as well).

Programming that is installed in a near-death state will exist at the most basic level, because the level of survival at that point touches the core of the being, regardless of whether the subject is well protected or not. The person who has experienced it may think that they will die if they try to break it. That they will be in a state close to death! That their heart will stop! I have gone through all of these fears and more while dealing with this type of inner programming and now I fight the residual terror it has left from time to time. The lies told in this almost unconscious state will be believed on a deep level, because the child who is experiencing it has a desperate need to believe the adults who literally hold his life and death in their hands. The child has been completely broken by the horrible programmed trauma and will adopt these messages as true.

This is why embedded beliefs and messages are so difficult to remove at this level. This requires excellent support, a safe environment and spiritual knowledge and insight, as the demonic stronghold will also be very serious. The help of a therapist who is knowledgeable about programming and a spiritual follow-up by people who know how to exorcise it will be a vital part of the therapy. The survivor who has reached this level of inner programming will have hit rock bottom. This programming will be one of the most integrated and will remain impossible to pin down on a conscious level unless there is deep cooperation, a safe climate and trust from the outsiders who help the survivor. This is also where faith in God, in His ability to heal EVERYTHING, even the most severe physical, emotional and spiritual traumas will make all the difference. This type of programming may require a safe hospital setting or an extremely safe outdoor environment, as fear can lead to panic and its externalization as it begins to drain away. A loss of reality can occur when the programming sequences surface and it will take powerful help to make the memories slowly emerge and be manageable. Medication will probably be needed to counteract a strong tendency to depression, a sense of loss, abandonment and betrayal that this type of programming involves.

There will be despair about the choices that have been made and a questioning of whether the memories can be survived. A compassionate attitude of encouragement can make a difference. Also very important will be reading scripture passages that remind the person of God's love and ability to heal, His care and promises of forgiveness. Disconnecting from this kind of programming is extremely tiring and requires a lot of rest and nutritious food. This is NOT the time to add external causes of stress. Allowing the survivor to vent their fear, reassuring them, praying with them and staying mindful will become life guides. Listening to his anger about what was done when he talks about the "sons of bitches who did this to him" will be healing and not rush him into premature or false forgiveness. The survivor will need to look at the trauma and wounds and acknowledge them and then discover that there is hope for survival of the memories of the embedded trauma. Providing good, non-mandatory experiences such as playing games, drawing, or taking a walk in nature will be healing. Outlets such as journaling and talking about feelings will be very important in the process of this type of programming.

I have just described one of the most traumatic programming that can be done in this group to a child or young adolescent. It can be overcome, slowly, with time and loving support and prayers. I hope that in telling this story I have not been too gory or too graphic, but that I have helped others to understand that this type of programming does occur and that the survivor of ritualized occult abuse has the need to overcome it.

EATING DISORDERS AND RITUAL ABUSE

"You're putting on a little weight," my stepfather remarked. I had come home from school that year and gained five pounds. He laughed at me when I came home. I was 14 and decided to start a diet. My aggressive diet was an immediate success because self-control and iron discipline had taught me from childhood to ignore my body's signals. I prided myself on my ability to eat only tiny amounts despite a nagging hunger. I lost weight quickly. "You're too thin, I can see all your ribs," my roommate said to me that year in school. "I'm worried about you."

"No, I'm too fat," I insisted. I looked in the mirror and saw someone who was overweight and needed to lose more weight to look good. Why couldn't others see that I was too fat? Several weeks later, my mother had to come and get me. My liver failed and I was hospitalized. I was 5'7" and weighed 90 pounds.

I kept saying I was too fat. I almost died from this disorder in my early teens and it would be years before I was anywhere near my normal weight. I never received therapeutic treatment for it because my parents didn't believe in it. Instead, my mother gave me a programming command, "eat, don't die" when I refused to eat. I was sent home. I shook for hours and finally grabbed the spoon and swallowed the soup. A young child who is systematically deprived of food and water to teach a lesson or to break him/her down and make him/her more accessible to programming messages will experience these long-term effects. Starving or starving are the primary elements of many Illuminati programming sequences inflicted on children as young as two years old.

The child will despair of eating once the deprivation is over and will associate eating with the comfort of the adults around them. Food becomes an additional area controlled by adults and trainers and the child begins to realize this early on. Although very young, the child cannot control how much food is allowed or if he/she is allowed to eat.

Cult parents, based on lessons learned at night, may also starve the child during the day or punish him if he dares to eat because he is hungry.

It is not surprising that many survivors of ritual abuse and cult programming are later found to have eating disorders.

There are several types of disorders. One of them is anorexia, where the person struggling with this disorder starves themselves to death. Anorexia has many causes, but a basic need for control and an underlying depression have been noted by therapists working with this problem, combined with a negative image and self-hatred. Self-hatred is polarized around body image and fatness. Some survivors with this disorder have confided that they starve themselves as teenagers to delay the onset of menstruation, delay breast development or other characteristics. Others with male alters wanted to have the flat chest that comes with being thin. And others starved themselves to ease the pain. Current research on anorexia shows that high levels of serotonin are associated with anxiety and feelings of distress, and some researchers have theorized that food refusal decreases this excess serotonin and effectively helps block these unpleasant feelings.

Another eating disorder is known as bulimia. This disorder is characterized by alternating bingeing or eating large amounts of food (often beyond the point of discomfort) in a very short period of time, and then evacuating the food. The evacuation is done by taking laxatives, by making oneself vomit, by taking diuretics, by excessive physical activity or by stopping eating after the binge. The person suffering from bulimia feels that he or she cannot control his or her bingeing and is ashamed afterwards.

Evacuation is the "punishment" for eating.

Janna struggled with bulimia for years. She never talked about it, not even to her sister or best friends. It started when she entered college after she gained weight. When she couldn't lose weight, she started making herself throw up after eating large meals. She also began using laxatives to "flush" the calories. "I knew I needed help," she states, "But I was too ashamed to talk about it." At age 27, her bulimia finally got out of control. It seemed to get worse when she was stressed, which was the case when she got a promotion to a responsible position. So much so that she began therapy to find the causes of the depression and suffering that had filled her life as far back as she could remember.

The third eating disorder recognized by experts is called binge eating disorder. Like bulimia, the person has an uncontrollable urge to eat and will binge to the point of abdominal pain in some cases. They store food and often binge in secret, eating very little in front of others. The person with this disorder is often in great distress because they feel they cannot stop. This person is usually overweight, and struggles with the problems that this brings.

Sarah hides donuts in her house and other favorite foods as well. "I once ate an entire cheesecake in one sitting," she admits. She hates being overweight and admits, "My doctor said this weight is killing me, that it's life threatening. I would give anything to be able to lose weight." But she also struggles with other feelings. "Being this strong makes me feel safe, despite everything," she confides. "I know men won't look at me." That's important to her, because she was raped by all the men in her family of origin.

Programming, sexual abuse, and trauma suffering within the cult all contribute to eating disorders that survivors struggle with. The reasons for dealing with an eating disorder are often complex and frequently unconscious. A child who was starved during the pre-school years may retain anxiety about food, stocking up on food in the house to ensure that he or she will never be hungry again. A child's alters who are constantly hungry because of these experiences may turn off the light at night and the survivor will wake up to empty a bag of candy or leftover desserts kept on the nightstand.

In some cases, despite the health risks (all eating disorders are dangerous), the survivor will retain an unconscious desire to punish his or her body and inflict disease or suffering on himself or herself. In others the desire may even go as far as a death wish and be part of a suicidal program.

Cindy is a 34-year-old intelligent woman and a model of beauty. Her heart is failing because she keeps starving herself.

"I know I can die from it, that I have to eat, my doctor keeps telling me," she shrugs and smiles, "It wouldn't be much of a loss, would it?" It's hard for her to believe that she's cared for and that others think she's a wonderful person, as she struggles with her inner messages of worthlessness and pain. "My mother used to hit me repeatedly if I ate too much as a child," she shares. "Maybe that's why I have a hard time today giving myself permission to eat."

Recovery from an eating disorder is often a long process that requires overcoming existing denial (the survivor often thinks there is no real problem, that friends and family care too much).

Therapy with someone who understands the underlying trauma and works with a qualified dietician can be invaluable. Understanding how the survivor feels about food, what shaped those feelings, and how they feel about themselves is part of the protocol.

If it is programming that is driving the disorder, it is also important to look at how it was done and why. Survivors have described many cases of "overfeeding to death" or "starving themselves to death" programming, especially if they try to leave the group/cult.

They can be helped by correcting a false body image, teaching them to love themselves and returning to normal eating patterns. The alters of a traumatized child can be reassured that the survivor will not tolerate starvation, and planning meals that give these elements an opportunity to choose their favorite foods can help limit nightly binges. Because each person is unique, healing will require dealing with their own individual issues. Healing is possible with the guidance of a trained therapist and with increasing cooperation.

A DAY IN THE LIFE OF A TRAINER

Warning: This article contains graphic descriptions of cult activities. Please do not read if this is a triggering risk.

Many people have written to me asking questions like, "When did you go to the meetings?" or "What happened to your children when you were in the group?" and even "How did you separate the cult activity from your normal life?"

This article will attempt to answer these questions and provide a better understanding of how dissociation works in a person who is active in a cult. This "day" is based on over 12 years of therapy and is a collage of many different memories of what my life was like seven years ago when I was still active in the San Diego group. I hope it will help resource people and therapists to better understand the severe amnesia gap between cult activities and everyday life, and that it will explain that a member of an occult cult practicing abuse can be a nice Christian in everyday life.

7 a.m.: I wake up tired, as usual. It's as if the fatigue doesn't let go of me, even when I go to bed early. I wake up with the alarm clock ringing and get up. I'm already dressed, because for over two years my husband and I have been going to bed fully dressed.

We laugh about it and agree that it saves time getting dressed in the morning. I am in the outfit of any American housewife: comfortable sweatpants and matching top, and tennis shoes. I dress more elegantly at work. I get my two kids up and make a simple breakfast of cereal and toast. Then they get ready for school and I drive them to the small Catholic school. I am a first grade teacher there; my daughter is in her last year of elementary school. I have a nagging headache that I force myself to ignore when I get to school.

8:45 a.m.: Class begins. I teach the first three grades of elementary school at a Catholic school my children attend. I used to homeschool them for several years. I was offered a replacement at this school when one of the regular teachers left and soon I was asked to teach full time. I love to teach and do well with multiple grade levels at once; I move from pre-K to subsequent grades, giving each one activities to do. My curriculum is prepared for the entire semester. I am found to be kind and patient, the children love me and I love them, despite the chronic headaches. They are sometimes intense at the end of the day.

3:30: The school day is over. My daughter has invited a friend home to play, so I remind them to buckle up to go home. I'm tired, but I also think it's important for my kids to have an opportunity to connect. Their tendency to withdraw into themselves sometimes annoys me and I encourage them to have more friends. We ride horses in the paddock behind the house. My son makes this comment, "Well, Mom, you're much nicer to me at home than when you're my teacher," and I laugh and tell him, "That's because I don't want to play favorites at school."

5:30 p.m.: I take the friend home. Dinner is in the oven. So far my day has been exactly like that of any person who doesn't suffer from dissociative identity disorder or belong to a cult.

That's because these are my daytime personalities coming through. They are sweet, caring, Christian and completely unaware of another life I lead. If you were to stop me at this point and ask me, "Are you involved in any nighttime activities?", I would have absolutely no idea what you were talking about. I was made specifically to look, act, and be normal on all levels during the day.

You could have followed me around all day and there would have been absolutely no indication that I was otherwise living another life. The only clue is the migraines and occasional unexplained bouts of depression where I can't stop shaking. Both of these things have dogged me all my life.

6:30 pm: My husband comes home and we all have dinner together. He and I are good friends, though distant in some ways: he lives his life and I live mine. We rarely argue or fight openly. I help the kids with their homework while he works on a client file.

7:45 p.m.: Phone call and when I answer, someone says, "Is Samantha there?" that's one of my code names and I get connected immediately. "Call back in a few minutes," I tell her. "Fifteen minutes," the voice says. I send the kids upstairs for their baths. 8:00 a.m.: Another call. "Samantha?" I change instantly. My voice becomes monotone and I answer in a flat voice. "Yes, what is it?" "Remember to bring the items we talked about last night," I am told. I then recite a code to this person, who is the head trainer, who makes sure I will remember his message. I hang up after him.

8:30 p.m.: I read a story to my children. They are very, very afraid of the dark, even at six and ten years old, and insist that we leave a light on in their room all night. As the evening progresses, they become more and more anxious. "Mom, I'm scared," my daughter says to me. "Of what?" I ask. "I don't know," she replies. She repeats this several times and I worry about my hypersensitive, anxious daughter. Inside, I know these fears are not normal and that there is something wrong, but I don't know what. My husband tells me that I worry too much and that our daughter is overreacting. I stay with the kids until they are asleep. This is our evening routine and I think it's the least I can do.

9:30 p.m.: I get ready for bed. I need ten to twelve hours of sleep a night, otherwise I am totally exhausted. How many times have I fallen asleep reading to my children. Just before I fall asleep, I tell my husband, "don't forget" and give him a code that will let us know we have to get up later. He replies in German that he will remember.

1:00 am: My husband wakes me up. He and I take turns waking the others. We don't need a bell, because our inner clock wakes us up. I'm in a jog, I fall asleep dressed to make it easier to get up in the middle of the night. I am finally me, I can now step outside and look at the world outside without the bars of my cage as I do during the day. "Go get the kids," he says in a low voice. I go upstairs and tell them, "get ready." They are up instantly, totally obedient, which is very different from the day.

Quickly, silently they put on their shoes and I make them get into the car.

My husband is driving, I am in the passenger seat. He drives with the lights off until we are on the road so as not to wake our neighbors. We live in the land of dirt roads and there are a few houses to be wary of. My job is to stay alert, watch for someone following us, and alert them if someone is coming.

Once on the paved road, he turns on the headlights and we head for the meeting. "I didn't finish my homework," my son says. My husband and I turn to him briefly, angry. "We don't talk about the day during the night, EVER!" we remind him. "Do you want to be beaten?" he looks uncomfortable, then the rest of the drive is silent, the kids watching out the car window as we silently glide to our destination.

1:20 am: We arrive at the first checkpoint of the military base. We pass through the back entrance and are waved through, the watchmen recognize our car and license plate.

They would arrest any unknown or unauthorized person. We will pass two more posts before arriving at the meeting area. It is near a large field on a very large Navy base that occupies dozens of acres. Small tents have been set up and temporary bases set up for night exercises. We come either here or to one of the other three meeting places three times a week. People chat and drink coffee. There are a lot of friends here because everyone is working towards the same goal. The work is intense and so are the friendships. I join a group of trainers that I know well.

"Looks like Chrysa is missing," I said. "I bet that lazy s...pe couldn't get out of bed." I am very different at night. I use words that would horrify me during the day and I'm mean and nasty. The others laugh. "She was late two weeks ago too," says someone else. "We may have to UNDO her," he jokes, but is partly serious. No one is allowed to be late or sick. Or too early. There is a ten-minute window for members to show up for meetings. If not, they are then punished if there is not a good excuse. High fever, surgery, or car accident are considered excuses.

Premenstrual syndrome, fatigue or a car breakdown are not. We drink coffee to stay awake, because even in the dissociated state the body protests being awake in the middle of the night after a day full of activities. I go to the locker room to change into my uniform. We all wear uniforms at night and we also have ranks, based on our position in the group and our service record.

1:45: We begin our assigned tasks. I brought the registers with me, the famous "object" that I was asked not to forget. I keep them hidden in a closet at home, locked in a metal box. These books contain the data of different "subjects" we are working on.

I go to the head trainer's office in a nearby building. I work with him, I am the second head trainer after him. We hate each other and I suspect that he would like to harm me, as I have made several cruel jokes at his expense. I am supposed to be afraid of him and I am, but I can't respect him either and he knows it. I point out his mistakes in front of others and he often tries to get even.

1:50: The room inside a shed-like building is set up for subject work.

It has a table, lamp and equipment. The room is separated from outside activities, so that others are not distracted by what we are doing here. The subject is here, ready to work on himself. There is someone else, a younger trainer who helps out and I tell her to administer the drug. We work on drugs that help induce hypnotic states and study the effects of these medications, in combination with hypnosis and electric shocks. We inject the drug subcutaneously and wait. In ten minutes the subject dozes off and his breathing slows down and becomes heavier, but his eyes are open, which is what we want. (I won't describe the rest of the session here, it's too painful for me to mention. I think human experimentation is cruel and should be stopped, but the group I belonged to practiced it regularly). We record data in the logbook throughout the session and I also have a laptop where I record information as well. We don't just profile the drug, but also the individual response of the person. We have very complete and thorough profiles on that person, started from childhood. I can extract a special profile that tells me everything about him: his favorite colors, what he eats, his sexual preferences, the techniques that soothe him and a list of all the codes that will cause him to respond. There is also a diagram of his inner world that has been created over the years. This is easy to work on and things are going well. At one point I correct the young trainer who starts something too soon. "You have to learn patience," I say, reprimanding her in German. At night, we all speak German, that language and English being the two languages of this group. "I'm sorry, I thought this was the time," she says. I then teach her the signs that the subject is ready. That's why I'm a head trainer. I train the young recruits, because after so many years, I know the anatomy, the physiology and the psychology. Luckily I caught this young trainer before she made a mistake; if she had, I would have had to punish her. At night mistakes are not accepted, ever. After the age of two or three, children are expected to perform well or they are bullied. This continues into adulthood.

2:35 a.m.: The session is almost over and the subject is recovering. The medication is working quickly and he will have recovered in time to go home. I leave him in the care of the young trainer and head to the cafeteria for a break. I smoke a cigarette while drinking coffee with the other trainers. I've never smoked during the day and coffee makes me sick, but here at night it's completely different. "How's your night going?" a friend, Jamie, asks me. I only know her as Jamie, it's not her real name, but at night we only use our nicknames. She is also one of the teachers at the school during the day, but we are not friends there. "Slowly. I had to correct another stupid kid," I said. I'm not nice at night, because no one has ever been nice to me. There is a "man is a wolf to man" and highly politicized atmosphere where the cruelest one wins.

"What about you?", I ask her. She makes a face. "I've had to march dirty kids," she says, referring to military exercises with children between 8 and 10 years old. They're going on every night, because the group is planning a possible coup. The children are divided into groups according to their age and different adults take turns instructing them. We chat for a few minutes and then go back to our "work".

2:45: This is a short session. It is the "harmonization" of a member who is a military leader. I take out his profile and review it before starting. The chief trainer and another trainer work with me.

The hypnotic induction is done quickly, and he remembers his program. We reinforce him with an electroshock and we control all the parameters. They are all active and well positioned. I sigh with relief. It was an easy case with no aggression against us. Afterwards, I comfort him and be nice. "Good job," I tell him. A small part of my stomach revolts at the brutality used to teach. He nods, still a little dazed from the session. "You should be proud of yourself," I say, patting his hand. We give him his reward afterwards, he will spend some time with a child. He's a pedophile and this is how he comforts himself after his session.

3:30 a.m.: We changed, our uniforms go into a special laundry basket before cleaning. I put my clothes, which were folded neatly on a shelf, back on and we all meet in the car to head home. My daughter comments, "I'm getting a promotion next week," she says proudly. "They said I did very well in the exercises tonight.

She knows that I and other adults will be at the ceremony honoring the promotions. I tell her I am happy for her. I am very weary for some reason. Usually I would be happy, but tonight, despite a routine night, it was difficult. I've felt a cold creep up on me lately and I've had bouts of terror. I sometimes hear a child crying inside, buried deep, and I sweat while working on children or adults. And I wonder how long I'll last like this. I've heard of trainers breaking down or not being able to do their jobs and I've also heard whispered stories of what happens to them. These are nightmares in essence and I am suppressing my anxiety.

4:00 a.m.: We get home and collapse into bed, instantly asleep. The kids fell asleep on the drive over and my husband and I take them to bed. We all sleep a deep, dreamless sleep.

7:00 a.m.: I wake up with the bell ringing, tired. I always seem to be tired and this morning I have a slight headache. I rush to get the kids up and get ready for another day of school. I wonder if there is something wrong with me as I seem to need more and more sleep and always wake up tired. I have no idea that the night before I was up living another life.

It may seem unbelievable to some readers that a person could live another life and have absolutely no idea, but that is the nature of amnesia. If the programming is done correctly, it is almost undetectable and the person will experience complete amnesia of their other activities. This is called dissociation and it exists in almost all members who are victims of cult abuse, such as the one I just described.

CHRISTMAS IN THE CULT

C hristmas is a time of warm family gatherings around the Christmas tree, the smiling sharing of gifts, and the excitement of sleepy-eyed children to see what Santa has brought while the adults drink eggnog and feast on joyful traditions.

But for a child raised in a Satanic cult, Christmas has a very different meaning. The day is taken up with the normal activities of shopping and entertaining and the family will be able to "warm up" during the day.

But at night things are very different. The child who waits during the day for Santa Claus and his gifts in the light of day trembles with terror at the thought of what is to follow at night.

The winter solstice is on December 21 and it is one of the strongest sacred days in the Celtic pagan tradition, as for the sect, the "New Year" starts after this date. Special ceremonies are planned to ensure a new year full of energy and it is the solar return of the lengthening of days (many occult ceremonies are also based on the veneration of an ancient solar deity). Moreover it is a Christian holiday celebrating the birth of Christ, despised by the occult group, and special ceremonies are scheduled to desecrate and distort the meaning of this day. For many occult families, the week of December 21–26 is filled with activity, as families are gathered together and there is no need to explain children's school absences.

The cruelty surrounding Christmas and the solstice is intense. Children are often subjected to abuse by cult members dressed as Santa Claus; or a parody of the nativity is played out with the result that "King Herod" succeeds in slaughtering the Christ Child (accompanied by the ritual murder of an infant). A child can be raped under the Christmas tree, and all the paraphernalia gives a new and macabre twist to this religious holiday.

Instead of celebrating the birth, the child raised in a family sect will experience Christmas as a time of horror and death. Programming is sometimes done, where images related to the religious holiday are implanted, and the child is told that seeing these images (such as a lit

Christmas tree or a nativity scene) will mean contact with the "family" or other trauma-induced messages.

Children (and adults) may receive gifts with hidden messages that remind them of past Christmases and traumas related to the "family" bond. A mockery of a sacred holiday is possible, but instead of eggnog and ham, the meal consists of repulsive foods.

These are just a few of the associations that occur in the disassociated alters of the child raised in a family cult, which is why many survivors feel a mixture of excitement and fear when the holiday season arrives. In addition, once the child grows up, the family members of the cult will go to great lengths to reconnect with him or her around the time of these religious holidays, to which all family members are necessarily expected to attend.

Panic and anxiety may occur in the adult survivor on anniversaries of intense trauma and ritual, and he or she may wonder why a holiday associated with togetherness means cowering in fear.

If the survivor understands for themselves where the panic is coming from and what the triggers are, they can find help. This will usually be done in therapy or by writing a journal.

If the survivor has stopped contact with family members, then he or she will receive a deluge of Christmas cards and gifts, and must be very cautious about this and aware that these items can be intense triggers. The desire to "call and reconnect" with family members will often be awakened by this and the survivor will need to work through this in therapy. The child's alters hold the most horrific memories and listening to them, allowing them to address their trauma and fears in therapy, through journaling and craft work can also help.

Creating new holiday traditions that are experienced as safe can also be helpful.

Some survivors will celebrate Christmas by doing things very different from their family of origin to help them convince themselves that they are capable of breaking free from all the traditions connected with it. And of course outside support and security will be best during this time.

Christmas is a particularly difficult time for many survivors. As adults, they may choose to let go of the traumatic meaning of the past and create a reassuring Christmas for themselves.

WHERE YOUR TAXES GO

I am writing this article to express some anger, but I can't help it. I am angry that my tax dollars are being used, and yours as well, to fund certain projects. I am taking the risk that my articles here on this site will be removed by writing this, but I cannot keep quiet.

There are CIA-led projects at Langley, Virginia. These projects are studies on techniques for various forms of mind control and how to easily coerce "subjects," drug them, hypnotize them, traumatize them or otherwise bring them under control and turn them into docile maneuvers who really think they are doing "good things" for their "country" or "family."

I should know better. I have been a victim of these brutal experiences and have experienced them on others later in my life.

There is a ton of documentation and evidence from both government archives and the internet that this stuff is really happening. These MK-ULTRA, BLUEBIRD, ARTICHOKE, MONARCH and other projects funded by your dollars have been and are still being used secretly to abuse and torture innocent children and then later as adults. The fact that there IS documentation available despite the monumental amount of papers going into government shredders shows the sheer mass of documents and notes that were kept and could not be completely eliminated from the public record.

We know from the PAPERCLIP project that Nazi doctors (you know, the ones who experimented on people in Germany during World War II) were brought to the US. While they seemed ostensibly there to help the US develop its technology, many of them also shared their knowledge of human neurophysiology, and were recruited to supervise future experiments.

Enough of talking in the third person. I want to share my own personal memories.

When I was 8 years old, at night, Dr. Timothy Brogan from George Washington University, my primary instructor and my mother would take me to Langley. I remember dark trees in the fields behind long buildings and that we always went to the same building.

Downstairs there were classrooms, which were used for training. I would sit in a group with other kids and watch movies about how to kill someone (we were forced to analyze these movies, questioned by the "teacher" about what the "subject" or "target" who was killed had done wrong, and how the killing was organized. We would analyze and discuss everything, including the direction of the wind, the type of weapon used, the scope used, etc.

Shooting exercises: there was a shooting range and we spent hours shooting. We learned how to take a gun apart and put it back together in ten seconds maximum. We were timed.

Training films: we were shown films on every topic imaginable, such as the "here are your leaders" films with a round table where the US Illuminati leaders would stand up when a leader entered the room.

The movies were sexually explicit, movies of violence, and movies about loyalty. We practiced blurring the lines (with someone following us) and how to follow someone without being detected. There was an isolation chamber in a room. It was not used for group exercises, but for special training sessions. Otherwise the room was sealed when it was not in use. Language training: different people came in and taught us various languages both with the class and individually. Sometimes my mother would sit and chat with her friend, Sidney Gottlieb, or with Dr. G. Steiner, a doctor who worked on this project with children. I don't know who the other children were or where they came from. Their families would go with them and come back for them afterwards, usually the mother or father or a family friend. The exercises ended at 4:30 in the morning.

Tulane Medical Center (where "The Institute" resides) was renowned as one of America's most advanced research facilities for mind control techniques and exploration of the paranormal, NDEs, and the endlessly repeated use of recorded messages. They believed that the near-death state would help embed a message or belief at the deepest levels of the unconscious and the "rebirth" experience (which created a new alter at a very deep level) gave a very, very loyal "subject." This was the case. The subject was terrified and told that if he ever disobeyed, he would be brought back to that state "at death's door," so there were not many who were "disloyal" under those circumstances.

The equipment that our tax dollars were used to purchase for these organizations operating under the cover of the government was very sophisticated: virtual reality equipment and the use of the most elaborate neuro-linguistic techniques. And people were taught how to use them most effectively.

The year I turned 23, I was a chief trainer in San Diego. At night I continued the experiments on others, under the supervision of Jonathan Meier and at the end of the day Colonel Aquinos, who was the regional director of our group.

And of course, at the end of each evening, we would download our highly encrypted data to the Langley data banks. At the CIA data center, we had to go through six levels of security passwords before we could get to the place where the data could be downloaded. They wanted to know the results of experiments everywhere, and there were strict protocols for reporting any unusual reactions, abnormalities, or new drug combinations that proved particularly effective.

I think the majority of the American public has no idea how their money is being used for certain government organizations. I also think that most people reading this would not believe that the CIA and a respected medical center could be the site of such experiments on the minds and psyches of children and adults (it was done on both). But it's the truth and I'm sorry, because it makes me angry that my tax dollars are going to subsidize abuse. My only desire is that one day this will be uncovered, brought to light, and the public will be able to scrutinize what has happened and is still happening, and that it will be stopped.

EASTER IN THE SECT

There are certain times of the year that are particularly difficult for those who have survived occult rituals. These are the "holidays" that correspond to rituals celebrated by occult groups. Although the actual rituals and practices may vary somewhat between groups, there are some similarities between them.

Easter is one of those times. In the group I grew up in, I was allowed during the day to live normally. Easter was a celebration of spring, the lengthening of days and the first flowers signaling the end of winter. I liked to play with the boxwood branches on Palm Sunday and look for Easter eggs around the church. And of course a little Easter basket with a chocolate bunny or lamb would appear.

But at night, the holy day was celebrated in a very different way. Much of the previous week was spent preparing for it (there was no school during Easter week when I was a child, in the years before the "spring break" that became commonplace. Most schools were closed for a week or even ten days during that week). The events of this period were quite painful, and included brutality, sexual abuse, and other rituals surrounding fertility rites, culminating at the end of the week with the parody of crucifixion. Often a child was chosen to undergo the crucifixion, a sinister caricature of the Christian celebration, and the adults declared that this ritual was an offering to debase the Christian tradition and to show its meaninglessness. I know for a fact that young boys were chosen for this ritual and it was horrible to see. A mock "resurrection" ceremony could sometimes be performed, but the resurrected person was not Jesus, but a demonic entity that would enter the person brought in a near-death state.

The spiritual roots of these ceremonies were created to allow the demon to pass into the participants, and to "seal" them as participants. Sometimes a golden chalice was passed around among the participants who drank from a cup filled with the blood of a child.

I am discovering more and more in therapy that I participated in these dark occult ceremonies as a child, such as those described here. These ceremonies allowed for the entrance of a demon, and one of the most difficult elements to dismantle in the programming done by the group was the hold that these memories, and the spiritual destruction that followed had on me. Part of my healing process involves letting go of what I suffered and replacing the horrific negative spirituality of my childhood with a belief in love, compassion, and forgiveness, the antithesis of the brutal and trying ceremonies I experienced. One of the most important tasks for survivors when they look back on these kinds of events (and anniversaries often bring back the memories) is to be able to heal and forgive themselves for participating, and to put in place a belief system that can supplement the negative. For me, that belief is Christianity and my hope is that others will find that comfort at this difficult time of year.

Realizing that very often the group makes certain things seem final can also be a great help. "You are doomed for life," they tell the children, or "You have accepted and now you are one of us forever." This is absurd. No contract is permanently binding, especially one created by coercion, and once a person has a choice, he or she may decide to break the spiritual contracts of childhood made under duress. The group during these times of celebrations and rituals tries to instill a sense of powerlessness and the feeling that "now I can never be free," but this message is absolutely false and plays on the fear of the little child. As an adult, on the contrary, the survivor has a choice and can choose to break these conventions and be free.

It's a struggle and I don't want it to appear easy. It's not and I still struggle with it, but it's worth it to break free of the hold that these ceremonies and demonic implications have on the survivor's life.

DENIAL AND DISSOCIATION

"... When denial is no longer necessary, neither is dissociation."

Once considered merely an annoying appendage in the diagnosis of Dissociative Identity Disorders, denial is now recognized as the "glue" that holds the dissociation in place.

The fact is that IDD would not exist without the need for denial. In other words, when denial is no longer necessary, neither is dissociation. IDD begins when severe and repeated childhood traumas causing intolerable conflicts in the young psyche, with extreme stresses, are resolved by a division into separate identities. This enables the person to repress the intolerable event so that other parts of him/her can live as if nothing had happened.

So-called intolerable conflicts arise whenever apparently vital beliefs are threatened.

These beliefs may relate to survival, safety, functionality, identity, morality, religious tendencies, or any other issue considered impossible to overcome. For example, most young children, because of their extreme vulnerability, believe that they cannot survive without a protective parent or caregiver. If, therefore, Dad violently hurts his children, this creates an intolerable conflict with the child's belief about the need for survival. The child resolves the conflict by creating a dissociative division in his mind, which allows him to "not know" about the event and thus be able to continue to believe that he has a protective relative and thus a means of survival.

The same kind of intolerable conflict occurs when the person is faced with an absolute need to function, yet is too upset by the impact of the trauma to do so, or when a person committed to high moral standards is forced to participate in "unthinkable" activities. Again a dissociation gives the person a way to be separate from the awareness of the trauma and thus enables them to do things as crucial as functioning normally or maintaining their moral identity.

Torturers, because of their knowledge of the mechanisms of dissociation, can deliberately create such conflicts in their victims whenever their agenda requires further splitting or absolute secrecy. They can do this easily by subjecting their victims to a trauma they think they will not survive, or by invoking intolerable emotions, such as life-threatening fear, humiliating shame, unbearable guilt, or by forcing them to participate in activities that conflict severely with their moral or religious beliefs.

Each of these situations will result in an intense need to deny the occurrence of the event, which will invariably create the dissociative wall desired by the torturer. Usually they make sure that the person is so deeply imbued with it that they can never get rid of it, which would mean that they would otherwise be confronted with reality or unbearable emotions. When the determining element that denial plays in the origin and maintenance of a dissociation is recognized, a profound change in therapeutic vision is possible. It is no longer necessary to precede the traumatic memories with the lived experiences. Instead, for true healing, it is necessary to address the need for dissociation barriers erected between the weight of the trauma and the maintenance elements of denial. This requires identifying and resolving the intolerable conflicts that seem to exist. This can be a very dangerous process, but it will focus therapy on the real issues that keep the dissociation going.

The survivor may abandon denial in successive stages. In the beginning, the idea of a multiple personality may be denied. When the reality of a division is finally accepted, the reality of all or part of the trauma may still be denied. It may be that one abuse by the persecutor is accepted, but not another, or that memories of sexual abuse are finally accepted, but not those involving Satanism.

The reality of the trauma may eventually be accepted in its entirety, but the possession of it may create resistance. In other words, the primitive identity in denial will accept that all these horrible things happened, but it will want to continue to remain separate from them. It is only when this core identity identifies personally with the events and their implications that the dissociative barriers can fall.

As this implies a major change, more for the basic denial than for the dissociation elements, the therapeutic orientation will play more heavily on these identities than before. Their threshold of tolerance must somehow be raised to a deeper psychological level. What was once seen as absolutely unacceptable must now become "appropriate".

Changing this perspective will require identifying, facing and rectifying many false beliefs. It will also mean facing horrible emotions and deep identity issues. The truth will only be revealed to the survivor through tremendous motivation, inner strength and courage. If you believe in God, however, know that he has promised to give grace and strength to accomplish all things.

Article originally appeared in "Restoration Matters," Fall 2001, Vol.7, # 1, online at www.rcm-usa.org. Diane W. Hawkins, M. A., reproduced with permission.

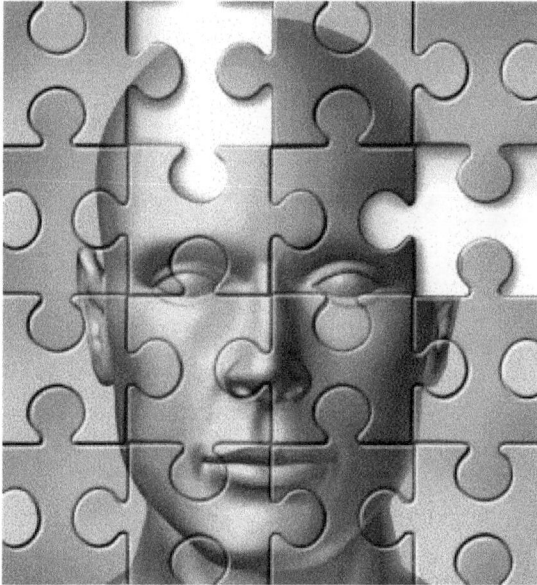

ALREADY PUBLISHED

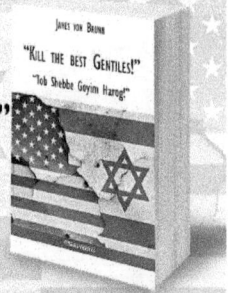
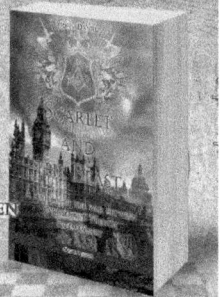
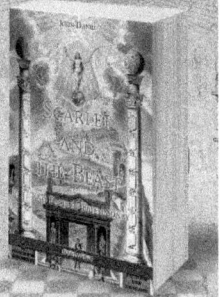

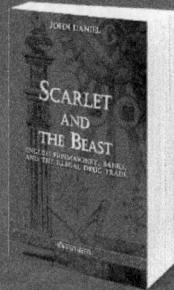

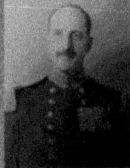

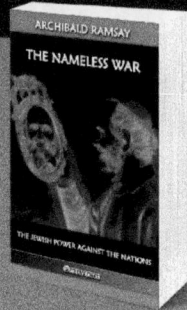

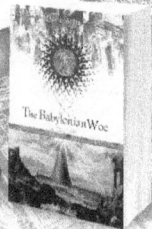

OMNIA VERITAS

Omnia Veritas Ltd presents:

FREDERICK SODDY

THE ROLE OF MONEY

WHAT IT SHOULD BE CONTRASTED
WITH WHAT IT HAS BECOME

This book attempts to clear up the mystery of money in its social aspect

This, surely, is what the public really wants to know about money

OMNIA VERITAS

Omnia Veritas Ltd presents:

FREDERICK SODDY

WEALTH,
VIRTUAL WEALTH
AND DEBT

The most powerful tyranny and the most universal conspiracy against the economic freedom of individuals and the autonomy of nations the world has yet known.

THE SOLUTION OF
THE ECONOMIC PARADOX

The public are most carefully shielded from any real knowledge...

OMNIA VERITAS

Omnia Veritas Ltd presents:

Fatima
and the
GREAT CONSPIRACY

This meant creating, or making, money out of nothing, being allowed to call it money, and to lend it to the public at a high interest rate.

This private syndicate acquiring a cast-iron monopoly over the supply and circulation of the money not just of England, but of the whole world...

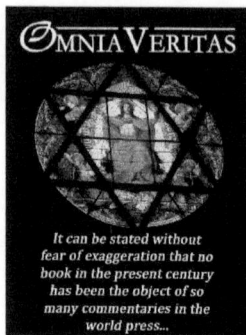

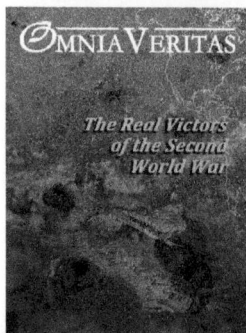

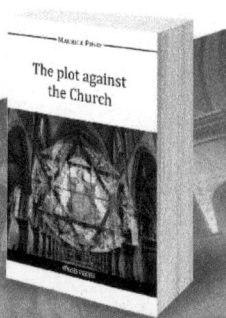

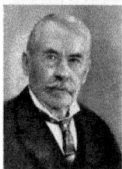

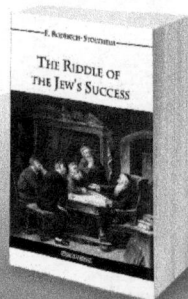

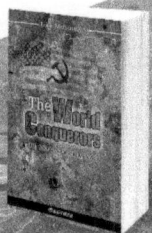

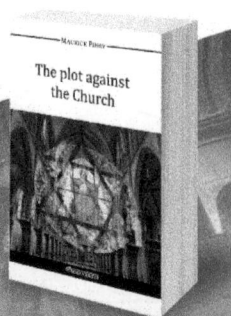

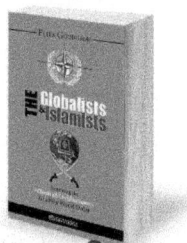